Praise for

What No One Tells You

"'No one ever told me about this!' is said by almost every woman during the often confusing experiences of pregnancy, birth, and the first year of motherhood. In this reassuring, accessible, and comprehensive guide, Drs. Sacks and Birndorf tackle common fears and questions—in particular, those that people may be embarrassed or afraid to mention. This is an indispensable resource for anyone who wants information that's both authoritative and comforting."

—Gretchen Rubin, *New York Times* bestselling
author of *The Happiness Project*

"Becoming a mom is magical. But it can also bring concerns and stress. In their loving and practical ┤...┤rf will be your trusted guides through ┤...┤times bewildering—experience."

—Harvey Ka┤...┤g
author of *The Happiest Baby on the Block*

"This book teaches mothers how to best care for themselves psychologically. I can't think of another book like it: written by experts who are both caring and authoritative and who can prepare new mothers for this tremendous identity shift and all the emotional changes that come up along the way. I wish I had a book like this when I was going through pregnancy and new motherhood."

—Christy Turlington Burns, founder & CEO of Every Mother Counts

Also by Catherine Birndorf

The Nine Rooms of Happiness:

Loving Yourself, Finding Your Purpose, and

Getting Over Life's Little Imperfections

(with Lucy Danziger)

What No One Tells You

A Guide to Your Emotions from Pregnancy to Motherhood

Alexandra Sacks, MD, and Catherine Birndorf, MD

Simon & Schuster Paperbacks
New York   London   Toronto   Sydney   New Delhi

Simon & Schuster Paperbacks
An imprint of Simon & Schuster, Inc.
1230 Avenue of the Americas
New York, NY 10020

First Simon & Schuster trade paperback edition April 2019

SIMON & SCHUSTER PAPERBACKS and colophon are registered trademarks of Simon & Schuster, Inc.

For information about special discounts for bulk purchases, please contact
Simon & Schuster Special Sales at 1-866-506-1949 or business@simonandschuster.com.

The Simon & Schuster Speakers Bureau can bring authors to your live event.
For more information or to book an event contact the Simon & Schuster Speakers Bureau
at 1-866-248-3049 or visit our website at www.simonspeakers.com.

Interior design by Ruth Lee-Mui

Manufactured in the United States of America

1   3   5   7   9   10   8   6   4   2

Library of Congress Cataloging-in-Publication Data
Names: Sacks, Alexandra, author. | Birndorf, Catherine, author.
Title: What no one tells you : a guide to your emotions from pregnancy to
motherhood / Alexandra Sacks, M.D. and Catherine Birndorf, M.D.
Description: First Simon & Schuster trade paperback edition. | New York :
Simon & Schuster, 2019. | Includes bibliographical references and index.
Identifiers: LCCN 2018044452 (print) | LCCN 2018046570 (ebook) | ISBN
9781501112577 (Ebook) | ISBN 9781501112560 (paperback)
Subjects: LCSH: Pregnancy—Psychological aspects. | Motherhood. | BISAC:
HEALTH & FITNESS / Pregnancy & Childbirth. | FAMILY & RELATIONSHIPS /
Parenting / Motherhood.
Classification: LCC RG560 (ebook) | LCC RG560 .S23 2019 (print) | DDC
618.2—dc23

ISBN 978-1-5011-1256-0
ISBN 978-1-5011-1257-7 (ebook)

For our mothers and the teachers,
students, and patients who have
mothered us along the way

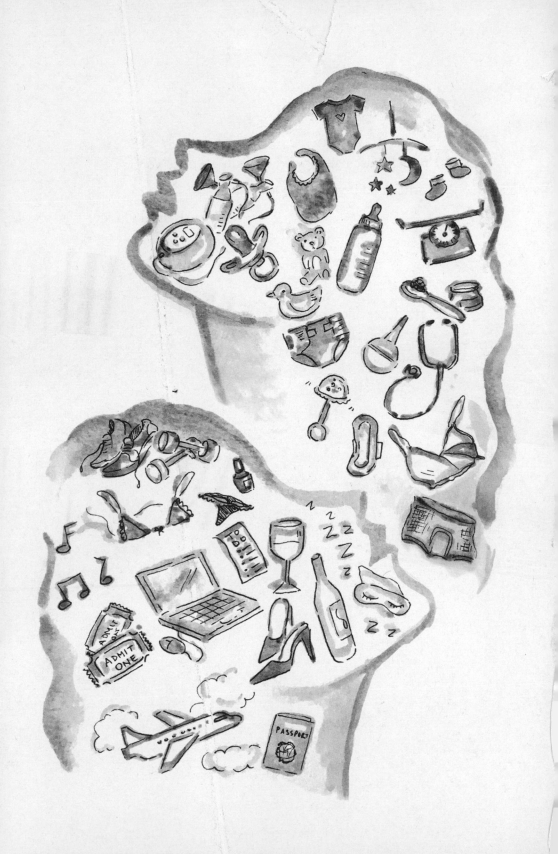

I remain fascinated by where you go once you are a mother, and if you ever come back.

—Rachel Cusk

Contents

- The psychology and social pressures of choosing a name.
- Handling weight gain and body image.
- How to stay sane while waiting for medical results.
- Sharing your news with a wider circle and at work.
- The good, the bad, and the ugly of pregnancy sex.

Chapter 3: The Third Trimester   81

Accepting and preparing for a significant change to your identity.

- How to become a mother without losing your self.
- Dealing with unsolicited advice, intrusive stories, and strangers touching your body.
- Financial planning for parenthood and its impact on your partnership.
- How to have a baby shower that will be meaningful for you—or no baby shower at all.
- The truth behind "nesting."

Chapter 4: Labor and Delivery   119

Facing one of life's most intense experiences.

- Mindful preparation for birth plans and birth classes.
- How to help your partner be a partner in labor.
- A primer on the hormones of childbirth.
- Deciding who gets to be in your delivery room.
- Meeting your baby and love at first sight—or not.
- Emotional recovery from physical trauma.
- The psychology of beginning breastfeeding.

Appendix 305

Figuring out if you need professional help and how to feel better.

- "The baby blues" versus postpartum depression versus postpartum anxiety versus matrescence.
- Risk factors and tips for preventing depression and anxiety.
- How to tell if you may have postpartum depression or anxiety.
- Primers on different types of therapists and therapies.
- Can you take antidepressants while pregnant or breastfeeding?
- What is reproductive psychiatry?

Introduction

Julie had dreamed for years about becoming a mother. It took months of trying, but finally, here she was, excited, grateful, and a bit nauseated. At an early doctor's appointment, she and her husband were relieved to hear that the screening results were healthy. Julie and her husband hadn't discussed whether they'd want to know the baby's sex in advance, but when the doctor asked, "Do you want to find out?" they locked eyes and agreed: "Sure, let's go for it." The doctor smiled and said, "Congratulations, you're having a boy!" Julie's husband squeezed her hand and beamed, but she felt her heart sink. Since the baby she had always imagined had been a little girl, she felt like she was losing that dream. *What's wrong with me?* she asked herself. *My baby is healthy, my husband is happy, and all I can feel is disappointment that I'm not having a girl?* She plastered on a fake smile, but as she gathered her things to leave the exam room, all she could think was: *Am I a horrible person? Will I be able to love my son?* Everything was going well, but Julie was spiraling, caught up in her worst fear: being a bad mom.

Julie wasn't a bad mom, of course. She loved her son, and once he was born, she would say that she couldn't imagine any other baby than him. But this wasn't the last time in her pregnancy or motherhood that she would be troubled by mixed feelings—about her son, about herself, about her choice to become a mother. And for Julie, as for many mothers, these ambivalent feelings sent up red flags. Anything less than joy and contentment, Julie thought, must mean there was something wrong. But that couldn't be further from the truth.

The expectation that babies bring ultimate happiness is not only unrealistic, it's dangerous. Our culture reinforces a story of motherhood that has left out doubt, uncertainty, and the bittersweet, and this myth has become hazardous to women's mental health. It's time to rebirth pregnancy and bring parenting down to earth.

We, the authors of this book, are reproductive psychiatrists: medical doctors who specialize in helping women navigate their emotions before, during, and after pregnancy. Because we listen to their stories every day, we know that most pregnant women and new mothers experience pressure to project an outward image of ease, when inside they're wresting with chaotic emotions.

Even if motherhood has been a lifelong desire, once it arrives, many women find themselves feeling lost somewhere between who they were before and who they think they should be now. And because many of our patients tell us that the only place they can be honest about their contradictory feelings is in a therapist's office, we know that too many women are ashamed to speak openly of these struggles for fear of being judged and labeled bad or ungrateful mothers. For most women, it's this shame and silence that's the real problem, not the experiences themselves.

Many women tell us they assume that having conflicted and confusing emotions means they are developing a mental illness. Of course, there are some women who need professional intervention. But over time, we've come to see that the majority of pregnant women and new mothers experience a natural emotional flux that falls in between bliss and the blues. Nothing as important as motherhood can be purely good or bad—it's far too complex.

Society seems to be invested in a "bliss myth," the idea that joy is the primary emotion of motherhood. But every mother will have moments of ambivalence, because she's always juggling between giving and taking. Since these conflicting feelings are rarely openly discussed, many women are left feeling that these struggles are their fault.

When women's stories deviate from this bliss narrative, they may feel alarmed and bury the experience, choosing not to share the uglier moments of motherhood with family and friends, and hardly ever on social media. Their stories are pushed deep down and left untold, and so the cycle continues.

Many of our patients tell us that they haven't heard sad or challenging stories about motherhood from others, so they are shocked when they have difficulty around common experiences like miscarriage, trouble breastfeeding, fighting with their families and partners, or simply feeling disappointed. A refrain that we hear again and again from our patients is: **"Why didn't anyone tell me it would be like this?"**

Sure, we all think we know the list of changes that come with pregnancy—you gain weight, your ankles swell, you have to pee all the time—but the reality is far more intense and abstract. Pregnancy is one of the most transformative events a human can go through, and dramatic changes to the body are never solely physical. Strange hormones will be coursing through your veins. Your role in your family will change—your relationship to your partner and to your own parents—as will how society sees you. It's a challenging journey, yet guidebooks have been scarce.

Most books about pregnancy are about having a good pregnancy, in which the goal is giving birth to a healthy baby. Most advice on early motherhood focuses on how to care for the baby, this strange and vulnerable new creature you're suddenly responsible for. Of course, women need this information. But pregnancy is not only the process of giving birth to your new baby—it's also the process of giving birth to a new *you*. And that kind of labor doesn't always feel good or happen easily.

We've all seen the Instagram or magazine images of the pregnant woman or postpartum supermom: a wise, efficient, gorgeous but modest multitasker who glows in her delivery room photo and laughs off the challenges of leaking breasts, dirty laundry, sleep training, an intrusive mother-in-law, and a grumpy, sex-starved partner. Her house is always clean, her hair is always done, and she's back in her skinny jeans just weeks after delivery.

Or maybe your image of the Perfect Mother is different. Maybe she's a savvy businesswoman juggling office and home life without breaking a sweat. Maybe she's a grounded earth mother, doing sunrise yoga and preparing organic meals for her family from scratch. Maybe she looks like your own mother. Maybe she's the exact *opposite* of your mother. Whoever she is, she's a perfect—and thus impossible—ideal. This is why the idea of the "good enough mother" (coined by the pediatrician and psychoanalyst Donald Winnicott) is so crucial but feels dangerous to many of us—it sounds like settling. The image of the Perfect Mother looms over us, even when we know that in other areas of life, striving for perfection only sets us up to fail.

Why didn't anyone tell me it would be like this? Well, we're here to tell you now. You shouldn't have to go to a psychiatrist to learn the nuts and bolts of how pregnancy and early motherhood impact your emotional life. This information should be as openly discussed and readily available as the advice in *What to Expect When You're Expecting*. After years of repeating this very information to thousands of women, we decided to write this book—at the risk of putting ourselves out of business.

This guidebook will describe how you may change in terms of your moods, hormones, brain chemistry, identity, and relationships when you become a mother. We'll take you on a chronological tour of the most important moments, from your positive pregnancy test through your baby's first year, and provide plenty of explanation and practical advice along the way.

We'll explore how to announce your pregnancy to friends having fertility issues, and why strangers may give you unsolicited advice. We'll discuss why some couples' sex lives fizzle and others spark during pregnancy, and the evolutionary biology behind the nesting instinct. You'll learn how memories may shape your experience of giving birth, and the most common reactions to being alone with your baby for the very first time.

Through the stories of women we have worked with, we will share how mothering is intergenerational: for better and for worse, your maternal identity is rooted in your mother's style, and hers in her mother's. You'll learn what to watch out for as you reexperience your own childhood in the act of parenting, repeating what was good while trying to improve upon what you want to do better.

We'll address competition: your friends and family, and even your spouse or partner, will be competing with your baby for your attention. Motherhood will also compete for the time, energy, and resources you're used to investing into your own life: eating, exercise, recreation, organization, sexuality, and work. We'll discuss how to navigate the shift in your role and relationship to all these people and places as well as yourself.

We'll teach you about attachment and how to understand your child's temperament, and provide advice on how to navigate relationships around child care. In an appendix, we'll discuss how to reduce the risk of postpartum depression and anxiety, how to know if you have it, and the science behind medication safety during pregnancy and breastfeeding.

Overall, this is a guide to taking care of yourself through pregnancy and motherhood, a period of life we call "matrescence." Try saying it out loud: *matrescence*. It sounds like *adolescence,* a well-described developmental phase and another time when bodies morph and hormones surge. Everyone understands that adolescence is an awkward phase. But during matrescence, people expect you to be happy while you're losing control over the way you look, feel, and relate to everyone around you. We're here to help you see the truth beneath those expectations.

A Note to Our Readers

This book is for opposite- and same-sex, cisgender and transgender, single and divorced, married and unmarried parents. We'll talk about vaginal birth, C-section, IVF, and donor eggs; we hope mothers via surrogacy, adoption, and many other paths find our postpartum chapters helpful. This book is oriented toward women who are physically pregnant. However, it is not meant to exclude anyone of any gender, parenthood story, or any family configuration. You can also look in the appendix for recommendations of other supplementary materials.

Much of the advice in this book is geared to the first-time mother; however, as every mother with more than one child knows, each pregnancy and parenting experience is different. If you're already a mother and pregnant or parenting with your next child, we think you'll still find much of the advice in this book helpful.

Though the psychological story of fathers and partners deserves its own book, this book may also be helpful for caretakers in many roles, especially in helping to understand and empathize with what your pregnant or postpartum partner is going through.

The patient stories in this book are derived from the combined thirty years we have spent learning from women. To protect privacy, the quotes used herein are not specific to any given patients but are our recollections of stories we have heard over and over that we have come to see as universal or emblematic and advice that we hope will be helpful to the majority of readers. While this book addresses the wide range of emotions women may experience during pregnancy and the postpartum, the anecdotes and advice may be weighted toward more emotionally challenging experiences, as our hope is that this book provides advice and support to women in need.

Finally, this book is not a substitute for proper professional care if you're experiencing significant distress that meets the criteria for mental illness or other medical issues. Please see the **Resources** for our recommendations on other communities and tools. And consider visiting us on social media to help expand the scope of the conversations begun here.

What No One Tells You

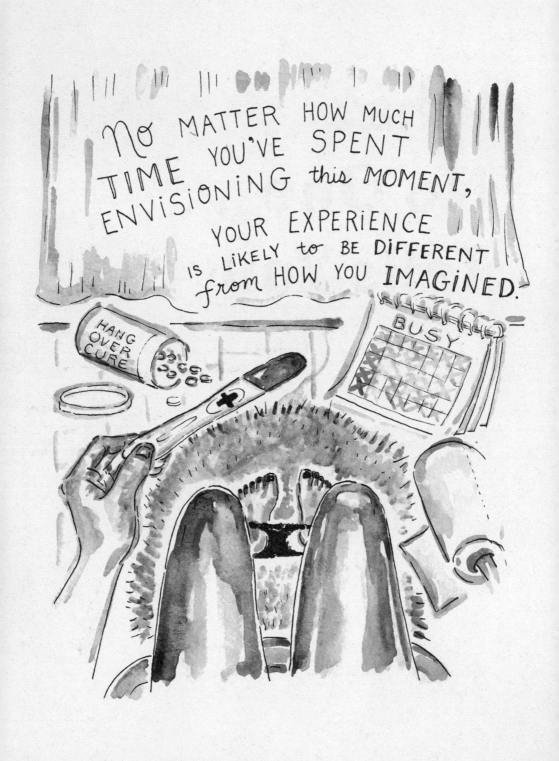

The First Trimester

Finding Out You're Pregnant

As the old joke goes, you can't be sort of pregnant. It's one of those biological experiences that happens in a sudden and life-changing way. While sore breasts and a missed period may give you a hunch, you can't be sure until you take a test. In those minutes of waiting for the result, you may feel terrified, excited—or a range of feelings in between. That plus sign is like a shooting star from another galaxy, a message alerting you to the future person growing inside your body but outside of your psychic solar system. This single signal marks two beginnings: your baby's, and that of your new life as a mother. You may have been pregnant for days or even weeks without knowing it, but as soon as you find out, everything is new.

If you're euphoric, enjoy your high. You might feel like you're the heroine in the victory scene of a movie you've been playing in your head for years. Especially if you've already faced months (or years) of negative pregnancy tests, you may even feel like you finally have been freed from purgatory.

On the other hand, it may take awhile for the news to feel real, and that disconnect can be disconcerting—especially if you're finding out early, when your body may not have begun to undergo any noticeable physical changes. Even more surreal is that this watershed moment is likely happening on an otherwise ordinary day. You might have errands to run, lunch with a friend whom you don't plan on telling, or work to return to.

No matter how much time you've spent imagining this moment, your experience is likely to be different from how you envisioned it. Even if you're intellectually thrilled, you may not feel the swell of spiritual glow you had expected. Your excitement may come later, in slow drips; perhaps you are even unconsciously titrating your reaction to avoid feeling overwhelmed. Particularly if you've lost an earlier pregnancy, or have experienced another traumatic loss in your life, it may take some time for you to let your guard down. And if you weren't expecting to be pregnant so soon (or at all), you might need to get through the disbelief and some tough decisions before you can feel like this is good news.

Maybe you got pregnant from a one-night stand and never saw

yourself as a single mother, but now you're considering having the baby. Maybe you're married but had planned to delay pregnancy until later in your career. Maybe your wedding is in six months and you've already paid for your form-fitting dress. Maybe you are the mother of two and thought you were too old to have a third. Maybe you've struggled through so many years of infertility that you're already in deep into planning another pregnancy with a surrogate (yes, this is a true story). The one thing we've seen time and time again is that your initial reaction is not a prediction of your future experience as a mother.

Even with a planned pregnancy, the first emotion many women feel is panic. Panic and excitement are often intertwined—they both make your heart race, and sometimes it takes awhile to figure out if the sensation is pleasurable or upsetting—but pure panic is an understandable reaction to the simple, sober truth: *Everything* is about to change. Panic is connected to our body's fight-or-flight response to immediate danger. The physical reaction of your heart pounding is part of an evolutionary strategy, a surge of stress hormones left over from when our ancestors needed energy to run away from predators hunting them on the savanna. It's human to panic when you find out you're pregnant, because the physical structure of your body and the emotional integrity of your psyche are about to undergo a profound overhaul. Even if you welcome the change, your life as you know it—at least in terms of time management and, for many, social and financial life—is "in danger."

It helps to remember that there's never a perfect time to have a baby, and no one is ever fully ready (even if she thinks she is). Having a child means taking a leap of faith—in your own body and abilities and, if you're partnered, in your relationship. Panicking because you're not sure you can do it, or because a part of you doesn't want to, is common—and, in our experience, unrelated to how you will eventually feel as a mother.

Certainly, many women choose to terminate pregnancies for reasons that are right for them. We've worked with many women who came to us for help because they were truly conflicted about keeping their pregnancies. Some decided that they didn't want to be pregnant, and termination was the right choice for them at that time. Others worked through initial feelings of apprehension to make a different choice. It's important to trust your feelings, but it may take some digging—with time or conversations with your partner, a trusted friend, or a professional—to figure out what's best for you.

One of our patients "accidentally" missed several termination appointments for her unplanned pregnancy. After some intense therapy sessions, she came to understand that she did want to be a mother but was just worried that she was too selfish to be a good one. She saw that her fears were tangled up in a history of anger toward her own mother, who had been emotionally neglectful toward her. This patient was ashamed about her drive for self-preservation and fearful that she was destined to repeat her mother's mistakes. But after talking through how she could protect some of her social and professional life in a way that would not be harmful for her future child, this patient decided that she wanted to move forward with the pregnancy. Now, years later, she's one of the most satisfied mothers we know, with a thriving daughter. Over time, she found a way to listen to her self-preserving instincts and also be a nurturing parent.

Preparing for Your Partner's Reaction

If you're partnered, and if this is a planned pregnancy, your partner may be the first person you'll tell. For some women, that's easy and obvious. Your husband may have been so involved in your pregnancy planning that he was standing next to you in the bathroom while you both prayed for the plus sign to appear on the test, ready to scream, "We're pregnant!" Your wife may have asked you to wait for her to get home from a meeting so that you could call your doctor's office together to find out your test results. Or, even if the news is a surprise, your boyfriend might naturally be the first person you call.

But whom you tell, when, and how is going to be different for every woman, depending on her personal style and the constellation of her relationships. Some women are used to going to the other women in their lives when they need to talk about "female stuff," from complaining about their periods to asking questions about sex. Telling your mom, sister, or best friend about your pregnancy can feel like a natural extension of years of "girl talk." It's not wrong to tell your partner second, but you may want to consider if he will be hurt or feel like his own privacy was disrespected if he's not the first person you tell.

However you share the news with your partner, be ready for her to have as wide a range of feelings as you do. One of you might be bursting to celebrate, while the other is preoccupied with miscarriage risk. You might both be freaked out, but your partner may react to that by wanting to wait a few weeks to share the news with others, while you can't wait to call your best friend. To find a middle ground, it will help to communicate about your different coping styles and support systems. Don't just tell your partner *what* you want to do—also try to explain *why*.

For example, if you've always told your sister, parent, or best friend everything (including secrets you haven't always shared with your partner), but your partner asks you not to tell anyone about the pregnancy yet, what will you do? How do you balance your obligations to your partner, your closest friends, and yourself?

One of our patients had learned through years of her marriage that venting about worries put her husband on edge. After sharing the news with him about her positive pregnancy test, she told him that she wanted to also talk to her best friend. She told us, "At first, my husband said he wanted to keep things private for the first month or two. My reaction was to fight back: 'This is my body. You can't tell me who I'm allowed to talk to about it!' But after some thinking, I found a logical way to explain to him why it was so important that I share the news with my best friend. I told him, 'Look, I love you, but we both know I like to vent, and my worrying freaks you out.' I was able to explain to him that being deprived of the outlet to talk to my friend was just putting stress on me and our marriage. He was able to see that I wasn't violating his privacy or choosing my best friend over him but just taking advantage of my full support system. And I made sure he knew I trusted my best friend to keep this private."

We recommend thinking about this first conversation about the pregnancy with your partner as the true beginning of your experience as a new nuclear family. Now that you're going to be together not just as a couple but also as parents, other relationships—even those with people as close as your parents, siblings, and best friend—will have to shift. You and your partner may experience this change as romantic, intimate, or intimidating. No matter how long you've been together, you've never shared a moment like this, and since neither of you is a mind reader, it's essential that you try to slow down and make some time for a quiet conversation, maybe one that is spread out over the course of a few days, and really listen to what the other has to say.

Sometimes you will learn that your partner is not on the same page as you about this pregnancy. He may become emotionally distant or cut off communication entirely. One of the most painful situations a woman may face is when her partner cannot—or will not—actively embrace his role as a father, and encourages her to have a termination she doesn't want.

If you find yourself in this situation—and your partner will agree to it—couples counseling with a mental health professional may help you both express and work through your concerns. Even if you're not going to stay together as a couple but you decide to keep the pregnancy, couples therapy can help you better communicate your expectations, which may later help with co-parenting.

One of our patients gave this advice after finding out she was pregnant with a man she had only recently started dating: "The clearer you can be with yourself about what you want before you include him in the conversation, the better. I was clear I was going to keep the pregnancy no matter what, even though I wasn't sure how the relationship would proceed. I told him I would be fully responsible for raising the child in every way. I realized that whatever I needed, I would have to go out and get myself. When I was having a bad day, I would remind myself how lucky I was because I was going to be a mother, and that didn't mean I had to stay with him."

If you find yourself in the situation of single parenthood not by choice, it's important that you start talking to family and friends early so you can begin building the community that will help you along the way. (See the end of this chapter for more advice for single moms.)

Telling Your Family

Your Parents

Many parents will be thrilled to hear that they're going to be grand-parents. But just because they're happy doesn't mean that there won't also be other layers to their reactions. Their exuberance usually involves sharing in your joy, and in celebrating their own life's goals to extend their family to the next generation. If your parents' lives are otherwise slowing down, a cute baby may be something to look forward to. They may also organize their identities around grand-parenthood to keep themselves busy and give them something to talk about with their friends.

Your parents' happiness for you may be mixed with their own sense of accomplishment, which can be challenging if they view the pregnancy more as something happening to them and forget that you're the mother at the center. No matter how grown up you are, you're still a child to your parents, so when you become a mother, they may inevitably experience some disorientation around this shift in the generational roles.

You may notice that it's painful for your parents to adjust to being the "second-tier" parents in the family, and for you to put your relationship with your partner and baby at the forefront. In response, your parents may, consciously or not, make other plans to busy themselves or make themselves feel important and generative. One patient told us that during her pregnancy, her parents decided to move to a retirement community and were increasingly unavailable, in terms of both geography and time commitment, since they were immersed in setting up their new home. If you notice that your parents seem uncharacteristically checked out, you may need to ask for their involvement more directly. They may be trying to stay out of your way to protect themselves from feeling like they're unwanted or hovering.

Some parents may weave between being intrusive and absent, especially if they're ambivalent about taking on the supportive but sidelined role of grandparent. Improved communication may help, but in many families, the decades of hurt or patterns of vulnerability may be too entrenched for one reassuring conversation to heal.

As life-affirming as pregnancy is, the birth of a baby is also about the circle of life—and the passage of time. Some grandmothers-to-be see their new status as signifying that they are now "old." If your mother remembers her own grandmother as wrinkled, gray-haired, and slow, she may not want to think of herself that way. She may react to your news by insisting that your child not call her "Grandma" or "Granny" but some other pet name. You may judge your mom for being vain and or a little petty—whether she likes it or not, she is becoming a grandmother. But her denial may be a way to cope with her own fear of aging.

And what about telling your dad? He may be overjoyed and supportive without being smothering. Or he may feel like you're "moving on" from him and your nuclear family, and he might express these feelings in unexpected ways. If he is a proud advocate of your career, he might tell you that you're abandoning your professional ambitions to have children now. If you plan to go back to work, he might say that he thinks you should be a stay-at-home mom. You can listen without reacting or agreeing if you're trying to keep the peace. Or you could take a risk and try to explain how these judgments make you feel and how your family planning makes sense to you.

From what we've seen with our patients, these intergenerational shifts may become fraught in the mother-daughter relationship, as you shift your primary identity from daughter to mother. You may not realize that you're on double duty, not only preparing to become a mother but also saying goodbye to your mother's role as the "primary" mother figure. No matter how close your relationship is with your mother, the adjustment can sometimes be challenging.

In navigating your new roles, you and your mother are renegotiating a new relationship. If you are used to agreeing on everything, new disagreements may be scary. At best, you'll be able to talk through tension to untangle miscommunication. Your mom may think that giving you (unsolicited) advice is showing love; you may have to explain that it feels controlling. She may experience your independent choices as a rejection, and you may have to explain that you're trying to feel more confident. She might even feel hurt if you hadn't told her you were trying, or she may feel left out from the decisions you've already made with your partner.

One of our patients told us, "My mom made so many assumptions about how involved she'd be in my pregnancy—she'd ask me when my next doctor's appointment was, and then put it on her calendar, assuming she'd come. We're close, but I wanted my husband to be with me at these appointments, and I knew he wouldn't want to share every moment with my mother. I had to have a really hard conversation with my mom, explaining, as gently as I could, what I wanted. She was hurt at first, but I texted her ultrasound photos and updates after every appointment, and that ended up helping her feel special. I just wanted her involvement to be on my terms."

What if you can't share this experience with your mother?

When your mother is absent—whether she has died, is ill, or is emotionally or physically absent—finding out that you're pregnant may surprise you with an intense new wave of mourning. If you no longer yearn for your mother emotionally, or have come to terms with that loss, this returned sadness may feel confusing, or you may have trouble finding its source. The intensity may take you back to the beginning of your grief, even if you thought you had left behind your "mother issue" long ago. We find that even if you're doing fine without your mother, pregnancy and new motherhood may turn up unexpected memories and longing.

If you were adopted, giving birth can conjure fantasies of a birth mother you never knew. This is natural, even if you are deeply attached to your stepmother, adoptive mother, or another mother figure. If you knew your mother but you no longer speak to her, you may feel sad that you don't have a good relationship but relieved that she's not there to interfere—and then you might feel guilty for that emotion.

It's easy to idealize someone who is not there. While it's lovely to think that your mom would have supported your every parenting decision and always been available to babysit, the reality would have been more complicated. She would have been human and flawed, as all mothers are.

It's okay to feel that not having your mother at this time in your life is flat-out unfair. Most women would rather a mother were there, warts and all. It's okay to feel sad and angry that she's not. Those negative feelings won't hurt your baby or your relationship with him.

Remember that just because your mother isn't physically here doesn't mean you can't welcome her memory in your child's life. You may want to write or record your memories and pictures of her to share with your child now and later.

If you are separated from your mother because of conflict, you may consider reaching out to her. It's always possible that a relationship can be repaired, and sometimes a child can be the reason. However, a joyous event won't necessarily heal old wounds or eliminate problematic behavior. If your mother's renewed presence causes chaos and pain, you may need to cut off contact again. As painful as that may be, you may be able to find some peace in knowing you tried your best to seek repair.

Almost all motherless mothers can benefit from having another nurturing maternal figure in their lives. If it's a friend or relative of your mother's, they may be able to share in your specific memories of your mother, and maybe in supporting you. But sometimes the most nurturing mother figures are not connected to your mother in any way. It's not required that these people be related to you, a woman, or older. What's important is that they are comforting and there when you need them.

Remember: Wanting or needing a mother figure in your life

doesn't make you needy or childlike. Most important, know that you're not alone. It may be helpful to connect with other motherless mothers online (see **Resources**) or through in-person support groups. You might also consider individual counseling or therapy to get the support you need to help you deal with any unresolved feelings.

Telling Your In-laws

When you tell your in-laws that you're pregnant, you may notice a shift in the intensity of their connection to you. The news might strengthen your relationship, solidifying your connection to them as family. But don't be surprised if their reaction to your news is focused mostly on their own feelings and fantasies. Your father-in-law might suddenly be interested in what you want for dinner because you're feeding his long-anticipated grandson (i.e., the boy he's expecting your baby to be). If your mother-in-law doesn't have daughters of her own, she might want you to share with her as much about the details of your pregnancy as you do with your mother. This may make you feel touched and eager to deepen your connection, or smothered.

If you feel that your in-laws are being intrusive and you're uncomfortable being the one to turn them away, this is a good time to enlist your partner's help in communicating with them. Even though you're the one who's pregnant, they are his parents, and you shouldn't have to shoulder their demands alone. **If you start setting clear boundaries now, you might discover that they will be better established and accepted by the time the baby arrives.**

Telling Siblings and Beyond

Whether or not you're the first in your family to have a baby, announcing your pregnancy may disrupt the established dynamics between you and your siblings. You may be hopeful that news of a pregnancy will improve your relationships—and for some, a new baby is a new opportunity for bonding. But it's also common to find yourself feeling disappointed when old dysfunctional patterns don't immediately evaporate. We encourage you to be patient with your siblings' reactions. This significant news can sometimes cause siblings to regress to a more childlike state, triggering old patterns of behavior.

Maybe your younger sister becomes preoccupied with also getting family attention for her wedding and gets worked up about the fitting for your bridesmaid dress, since you'll be pregnant at her wedding. Maybe your older sister is supportive but says that you're being "silly" when you ask if she's upset because she's had fertility issues. Maybe your spaced-out younger brother doesn't return your voice mail, and you have to share your personal news via text message, which may leave you feeling cold.

Even if you're not surprised by your siblings' behavior, you may still find yourself wanting them to respond in other ways. Remember that your siblings have nine months to get on board, and once the baby feels more real to all of you, they may become more invested in their status as aunts or uncles. **As with your parents, you may have to meet your siblings where they are emotionally, wherever that is right now.**

Ask Yourself Before Sharing the News

Your doctor may give you more guidance about your specific circumstances, but since most miscarriages take place in the first trimester, many women decide to keep their news relatively private until the higher-risk time frame has passed. There are no firm rules here, but the following is a list of questions we encourage all our patients to consider about sharing the news in your first trimester:

- Is everyone I'm considering telling about my pregnancy also someone I would be okay knowing if I had a miscarriage?
- Am I someone who feels best when connected to my support system, so even if the miscarriage risk is currently higher, I would want everyone I love to be able to support me, especially if I had a miscarriage?
- How does my partner feel about my telling this person?
- If my partner wants to keep the news private, might that be positive for our relationship and setting up boundaries for our future family?
- If I tell this person, will they keep the news private or might they gossip (with other family, friends, coworkers)?

- I may want to tell people at work by way of explaining why I'm tired/not drinking/rushing to the bathroom, but would sharing the news this early also compromise my privacy? Is there one trusted person I can tell, or can I give myself permission to keep this private without feeling like I have to defend myself for my body's demands?
- Am I ready to deal with the questions that may come with the news (Are you moving? Are you going to stay at your job? Are you going to raise the baby a certain religion?)?

Finding Your Blind Spots

As motherhood approaches, you'll find yourself not only renegotiating your relationship with your parents but also reevaluating your understanding of them and the ways they have influenced your life. How do you feel when you compare yourself to your mother? Do you already feel like a failure and ashamed for your perceived flaws? Do you see how her mothering has helped influence the woman you are today? Or does thinking about this make you well up with sadness, acknowledging how profoundly disappointing your mother was to you?

Maybe you saw your mother as perfect through your young eyes. She always seemed to know just what to do or say, and made you feel warm and safe. If you grew up with a mom like this, consider yourself lucky: You have a model to follow. Once your baby is born, you may find yourself rocking him to sleep, cooing the same lullaby that once made you feel so soothed. Even if he is crying and refuses to settle down, you may be calmed by knowing that following your mom's example will lead you in the right direction.

The downside of this type of legacy is that your mom may loom as an impossibly perfect standard. Rather than comparing yourself to her flawless memory, take the opportunity to ask your mom what the early years of parenting felt like to *her*. She'll probably admit that she was winging it and doubting herself a lot more than it seemed.

On the other hand, most of us can remember moments from our childhood when we promised ourselves that we would do better than our mothers. Maybe it was the time she scolded you for something in front of your friends, or left you waiting at school until you were the last kid. The first trimester isn't too early to start seeing the challenges of motherhood as a chance for forgiveness for both her and yourself. If you arrive too late for a visit with your practitioner because you didn't leave enough time and got stuck in traffic, maybe you can consider both yourself and your mother in a gentler light.

There may also be times when you'll catch yourself acting like your mother in a way that makes you cringe. Maybe you're irritable, criticizing your partner. You explode at him for something small, and you're not quite sure why you're feeling so volatile. You're so mad, you're even mad at yourself for being mad at him.

When you cool off and think about what set you off, you may realize that the fight you were having reminded you of the way your mother criticizes your father. As a little girl, you used to lock yourself in your room when they were fighting, you hated it that much. So why would you repeat the same behavior that disturbs you from your own past?

If you find yourself repeating a painful pattern from your own childhood, you may be encountering one of your psychological "blind spots." We call them blind spots because they are like the places in your rearview mirror that you can't see; thus, they can cause "accidents" because you're not aware of the hidden danger. The technical term for blind spots is "unconscious conflicts." They are unresolved feelings from your past that you have buried deep down below your awareness because they are too difficult to look at directly.

The mind makes blind spots as a way of defending against memories and feelings that are too painful to revisit. This protects you from being overwhelmed by your emotional scars in the everyday. That is helpful until something in your daily life triggers a reminder of a blind spot. This can be as simple as how becoming a parent easily places you in situations that remind you of your own parents.

Another way of thinking about blind spots is that they are "portals" to your past. When you're inside one of these portals, you're accessing the painful feelings you had in childhood, and you can easily lose perspective about the here and now. That's why it's important to learn about your blind spots before your child is born and, ideally, notice when they come up in your parenting.

In psychology, we talk about learning how to see your own blind spots as part of developing an "observing ego." This is the ability to step outside yourself (especially if you're behaving in ways that you don't want) and reflect on what you're feeling. With an observing ego, you can think about *why* you might be falling into this undesired pattern before you start behaving in ways that you'll later regret. In other words, it's learning to identify how you're feeling before you react impulsively, and getting to know your blind spots well enough so that you can sense them even if you can't exactly see them clearly.

For example, if you feel anxious at all your doctor's appointments, you can take a step back and think about what the appointments trigger for you. You may realize that you worry about your health to an irrational degree because, for example, your mother was seriously ill during your childhood. Rather than becoming consumed by irritability, or going into unhelpful control-freak behaviors at the appointment, your wise observing ego might be able to inform you: *That tightness in your chest? It's the tension you always feel around doctors. Rather than becoming mean or bossy because you're feeling so out of control, why don't you try explaining to your partner and doctor that you're feeling scared. Or just closing your eyes and reminding yourself that it's just a feeling from your past, and you're safe here and now.*

During pregnancy, your intense emotions and regrettable

behaviors may provide some clues about blind spots from your childhood. It takes a lot of self-examination to develop an observing ego, and most people benefit from working on this with a therapist, because they are trained to help you learn how to identify your own blind spots. In therapy, our job is to help you recognize these portals and feelings so you don't repeat patterns of behavior that you're trying to avoid. When we can bring these unconscious feelings into our conscious mind, we have a chance to work through them and gain more agency over how our feelings impact our choices.

Managing Worry and Balancing Control

Much of the emotional distress that women tell us they feel in the first trimester is motivated by a paradox: On one hand, you have new rules about what you can and can't eat and drink to make sure your baby is healthy. On the other hand, you're told that in the early weeks of your pregnancy, the risk of miscarriage is at its highest, and that if you're going to miscarry, *there's probably nothing you can do about it.* Balancing these two facts is psychologically exhausting.

Most women fall somewhere in between cautious optimism and painful pessimism as they move through the first trimester. While worrying about miscarriage is totally normal, and some pregnancies do end in miscarriage, the odds are most likely in your favor for a healthy pregnancy.

If you are feeling worried about doing something that will cause a miscarriage—or you're replaying cocktails you consumed before you knew you were pregnant—know that most miscarriages are not caused by anything you did wrong or could have controlled. The biology of early pregnancy has evolved over millennia, and embryos are pretty resilient. Especially in the first trimester, their development is most influenced by their genes, not their environment. Many first-trimester miscarriages are due to a genetic problem—not necessarily a permanent issue with your or your partner's genes but a mutation on the sperm or egg that happened to form this embryo. In this situation, the code programming that embryo's growth goes awry, and may lead to a nonviable pregnancy. It's a biologic event, and no one's fault.

If you've had a miscarriage (or miscarriages) before, your heart may still be somewhat in the past during this pregnancy, remembering that other loss. No matter how long it has been, you may not want to let your guard down and allow yourself to feel happy, at least not yet. **Fear of a miscarriage may also be tied to other losses from your past, such as the death of a parent or a prior medical illness or trauma of your own.** Or you may simply be a person who anticipates the worst and finds in worrying a sense of control, as if you're planning for the worst by dwelling on it.

What If I Miscarry?

There are many different reactions to miscarriage, and none of them is wrong. For some women, miscarriage is painful but doesn't leave a lasting wound. They recover physically and gear up to try to get pregnant again. Other women feel the loss profoundly and mourn the potential child as if it had been born.

If you miscarry, it won't necessarily mean that your body is defective or that your next pregnancy won't be healthy. It won't mean that you're not meant to be a mother. While blaming yourself may give you a momentary feeling of making sense out of this mysterious disappointment, in the long run, it's not going to make you feel better.

Whatever your experience, it's important that you not become isolated. If your friends and family don't understand your reaction to losing this pregnancy, try not to judge them—or yourself—for it. Consider reaching out to local and online support groups that can give you the support and validation you need at this time (see **Resources**).

Pregnancy is the first time many of us confront the reality that no matter how much we try to control our body, it can disobey us. At the same time, healthy behaviors can go a long way to sustaining wellness, and there are concrete things you can do to increase your chances of a healthy pregnancy. For example, if you stay within the medically recommended weight guidelines, you may be able to reduce your risk of gestational diabetes. (But even if you drink kale smoothies all day long, you can still develop preeclampsia.) The profound randomness of pregnancy outcomes can feel like a cruel joke.

You'll be given lists of foods not to eat, substances to avoid, vitamins to take, exercises to practice—reorienting much of your life and behaviors around striving for a healthy pregnancy. This may feel intense, and it is just your first taste of a lifetime of balancing your own needs with what is best for your family. It's an introduction to the many emotional contradictions that you'll face as a mother.

No matter how committed you are to maximizing your baby's health, you may also feel a pang of longing when you have to pass on your end-of-the-day glass of wine—your preferences are being subordinated to the needs of the creature growing inside you. You may decide that giving up your second cup of coffee is making it impossible to focus at work, so you'll talk to your doctor about an acceptable modification. You may be grumpy about nine months without soft cheese. Don't feel bad for those urges and longings— it's natural to want to continue to enjoy your life in your usual way.

Not every pregnancy rule is going to chafe, though. For some women, pregnancy is a compelling incentive to create a healthier life. Who among us couldn't use some motivation to exercise more regularly, eat healthier food, or drink more water? We've seen patients stop smoking overnight after years of trying to quit. Many pregnant women suddenly want to go to the gym, cut out alcohol, or get more sleep, easily adopting new healthy habits that would've been unthinkably challenging before.

But that doesn't mean you have to be an angel. If you had a couple of drinks on the night you conceived, remember that you're probably the rule rather than the exception. Most women find out they're pregnant after they miss a period. Racking your brain about your behavior in the previous few weeks is a common source of stress. The reality is that many pregnancies are (at least consciously) unplanned, so that means many pregnant women don't start taking prenatal vitamins and all the rest until they get that positive test. If you find out you're pregnant later in the first trimester, or you're concerned that your past behaviors have affected your baby, ask your doctor. Be completely honest with her about anything you did that concerns you so she can care for you appropriately. This applies to lifestyle choices as well as medications. If you are taking psychiatric medications, whether or not to continue them during pregnancy is a complex subject. We address it in detail in the **Appendix**.

With so much out of your control, it can be tempting to become extremely strict about what you *can* control, but this can lead to an unhealthy all-or-nothing mentality—as if a normal level of being good isn't good enough. If you find that you're berating yourself when you don't make a "healthy" choice (you ate a bag of candy instead of an apple), remember that no single behavior will determine the outcome of your entire pregnancy.

Worry vs. Anxiety

We think of "worry" and "anxiety" as essentially the same thing. The words describe emotions, like happy or sad. Both "worry" and "anxiety" describe common reactions to situations and events over which we feel unsafe or out of control. We also use the word "anxiety" when we're describing a medical condition. "Clinical anxiety," also known as an "anxiety disorder," is the medical name for when anxiety and worry become so intense or pervasive that you have trouble functioning in daily life. Anxiety disorders should be addressed with a mental health professional (more on that in the **Appendix**). But in everyday language, "anxiety" and "worry" are used to describe common, healthy—if unpleasant—emotions. We'll use them interchangeably in this book.

Sometimes when we are plagued by worried thoughts, we can talk ourselves out of them. Often these types of thoughts take the form of questions we ask ourselves: *What if breathing in that dust from the construction site I just walked past makes me miscarry?* Instead of spiraling deeper and deeper into catastrophic worries, write down your questions and bring them to your next obstetric appointment or call your doctor to ask. You will likely get a reassuring reality check. **We caution against googling, because you never know if an** internet source is reliable, and inaccurate information can raise your anxiety level.

How to Reframe Your Worries When They Feel Out of Control

Worrying can quickly become a problem when wondering "what if" leads you to unlikely worst-case scenarios. Because of their vividness, they can start to feel like a real threat. When a thought feels sensible or "true" but isn't actually rational, that's called a "cognitive distortion." Here's an exercise that can help you build perspective in your thinking and aid in getting worry under control:

1. **Write down your worries and your feelings about them:** *It's awful that I slept through my yoga class. I'll never be able to motivate myself again. Or, I ate half a pizza and didn't have any vegetables yesterday, I'm going to give myself gestational diabetes, and my baby's going to be sick.*

2. **Assess what you wrote and reframe by eliminating the judgment—just detail the facts as best you can:** Looking at what you've written, you may see lots of worst-case scenarios and catastrophic results. Try to rewrite your worries with a more likely, less extreme outcome. *I slept through my yoga class, so I may be less flexible the next time I go, but I can regain that flexibility. Or,*

27

I ate half a pizza and didn't have any vegetables yesterday. I might have a bit of a stomachache later, but I'll get back to my healthy eating tomorrow.

3. **Challenge yourself to frame your worry optimistically:** Consider a possible benefit that your "bad" choices brought you. Write those out, too: *I slept through my yoga class, and I feel so much more rested now.* Or, *I ate half a pizza, and it was delicious.*

The point of this exercise is to help you see that any one regrettable choice doesn't need to define or condemn you; that worst-case scenarios are usually unlikely; and that rather than beating yourself up, you can simply make a different choice next time.

The tension between the rules you're being told to follow and your inherent lack of control can be exhausting. It's important to be aware of the emotional toll of this experience and to make sure it doesn't take over your life. As hard as it is, you'll have to accept a level of uncertainty. We've seen women create irrational rituals—like unplugging the microwave to protect against miscarriages—to give themselves a sense of control over the uncontrollable.

Growing a human is hard. If your quirks or rituals are making your emotions easier to navigate, then be as "weird" as you need to be. Quirks aren't a problem until they start interfering with your daily life.

Washing your hands twice after you go to the bathroom isn't a big deal. If you wash them until they're cracked and bleeding, that's a problem.

One of the biggest lessons of pregnancy (and, later, mothering) is the need to accept what you can and can't control. If you find yourself trying to control *everything*, remember that, as scary as the thought may be, perfect rule-following does not mean a perfect outcome. Nine months of rigid strictness will not guarantee you a healthy baby—and may make you feel confined and deprived, which, for some people, can lower mood and raise anxiety.

A Hormone Primer

Remember the intense emotional reactions you experienced as your body went through the changes of puberty? Estrogen and progesterone, the same hormones that rocked you then, are once again triggering changes across your nervous system and body, along with other hormones that are working to support a healthy pregnancy.

Not everyone reacts in the same way to those changes. You may get morning sickness or feel like you're on an emotional roller coaster, or you may feel amazing. You could feel spaced-out or suddenly find that you're able to focus like a laser on everything from a report at work to cleaning behind the fridge.

Here's a brief primer on the major hormones of pregnancy, and how they may affect you emotionally. They all interact, so you can blame or celebrate them all at once if you prefer.

Estrogen: This is a big one, especially in the first trimester. Estrogen may interact with neurotransmitters (brain chemicals such as serotonin and norepinephrine), which can make you feel better or worse. As estrogen production revs up, your emotional shifts may become more dramatic and this could result in mood swings. (This is also an issue postpartum, when estrogen levels dramatically drop.) It's not the exact amount of estrogen but the sudden changes in levels that cause some women to experience mood swings.

Progesterone: This hormone relaxes your blood vessels and can lead to lower blood pressure, which could make you feel light-headed and dizzy. It relaxes different types of muscles in the body, including those in your gastrointestinal tract, which may lead to the distressing experiences like reflux. It can also make you drowsy, relaxed, irritable, or moody.

Human chorionic gonadotropin (HCG): This is the hormone that starts telling your body you're pregnant; pregnancy tests work by detecting the rise in the level of HCG. While the exact cause of pregnancy related nausea and "morning sickness" is unknown, it may be related to HCG.

Oxytocin: Known as the love hormone (but far more complicated than that), oxytocin both stimulates and is stimulated by intimacy. That means it can make you want to cuddle your partner (and, later, your baby); also, skin-to-skin touch may make you produce more of it. This hormone can make you feel sleepy, sentimental, and nesty.

Corticosteroids: These "stress hormones," which include cortisol, do many things, including suppress your immune system, and catching a cold during pregnancy is no fun. There's a good reason your body does this. Your baby's DNA is (unless you're using a donor egg) 50 percent yours and 50 percent from the sperm that fertilized your egg. When you get pregnant, your body sees the foreign DNA as a threat and would attack it if it weren't for this weakened immune system. These hormones may also rev up your fight-or-flight system, making you feel edgy or on guard. This experience may also contribute to feelings of anxiety or irritability.

Insulin: Your body produces insulin to break down food for energy. When you're pregnant, your body also uses insulin to help the placenta become more efficient in absorbing the energy it needs to feed your baby. Sometimes, fluctuations in insulin levels may cause a drop in your blood sugar levels, which may leave you feeling hungry, fatigued, sluggish, or spaced-out.

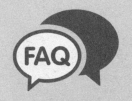 The following are some of the most common questions women ask us in their first trimester:

If I went through fertility treatments, how will that affect my outlook on the pregnancy?

Just because you're physically pregnant doesn't mean that your emotions aren't still recovering from the infertility experience. If your fertility treatments have included months or years of medical intervention, you're hardly starting from square one. You may already be exhausted, nauseated, or bloated because of the drugs you've been cycling through, especially if you've had multiple rounds of egg retrieval or in vitro fertilization (IVF.) You may already be fed up with restrictions on your travel or exercise that began even before pregnancy. You've already sacrificed emotional and financial resources and may feel spent at the beginning of your pregnancy—the way many women feel at the end.

On the other hand, you may have already begun some emotional growth that pregnancy often demands, like having to come to terms with what your body can or can't do. You may have matured in your ability to tolerate feeling out of control, which will benefit your future parenting experience.

There is a wide range of natural psychological responses to finding out you're pregnant after fertility treatments. Some women are able to leave behind their infertility experience when they walk into the obstetrician's office for their first-trimester appointments. Others struggle with celebrating their pregnancy or feel cut off from their happiness. Some women who have faced fertility disappointments aren't able to embrace their pregnancy until after the first trimester, when the risk of miscarriage decreases. Others still brace themselves for bad news until they can hold their healthy baby in their arms.

If you conceived using a donor egg or sperm, you may worry over how you'll feel about your baby because he may not share some or any of your or your partner's genetic material. Let us remind you that even if you and your partner conceived traditionally and without intervention, there would be no guarantee that the baby would be similar to you in any particular way. Biology doesn't promise that you'll pass on your partner's calm temperament or your green eyes. **Genes may make people biologically linked, but they do not make a family.**

We encourage any mother who is feeling concerned about using donor eggs or sperm to address their fantasies (and fears) that their parenting experience will feel unnatural or inferior. Regardless of biology, there's really no way to know what your parenting experience is going to feel like until the time comes. This seems to be true for most families, even those who conceive without any reproductive assistance. Furthermore, science still doesn't really know how much of a child's behavior is nurture versus nature. Parenting is defined by your caretaking, and the emotions in your heart. You, your child, and your relationship are so much more than your biology. Please see our **Resources** section for more information.

What should I expect from pregnancy with twins?

One consequence of conceiving through fertility treatments may be a higher incidence of twins and other multiple births. You may have anticipated conceiving more than one baby at a time, or multiples may be what you were hoping for.

If you haven't used any reproductive technology, finding out you're having twins may come as quite a shock, even if multiples occur in your or your partner's family. If your first thoughts are: *How the hell are we going to care for them or afford this?* or *I wish we were only having one*, we can promise that you're not alone.

Don't punish yourself if your reaction isn't what you think it should be, and try not to push the feelings down. You're not rejecting your babies, you're upset because you haven't yet figured out how it's going to work. Many of us don't react well to unexpected news, even if it's welcome. You just need some time to absorb this new information and get used to the idea. You'll have time to educate yourself, figure out a work/financial plan, and put a support team in place.

Moms of multiples are also often concerned that they won't be able to bond with two or more babies at the same time, or that they won't be able to meet the infants' emotional needs. This is completely understandable. Even if you have help caring for your babies (and we hope you will), you won't always be able to satisfy both children at the same time. This may make you feel like you're constantly failing because there's no way to give each baby enough attention. However, it's good to remind yourself that many mothers take care of multiple children (even if they weren't all born at the same time), and most families find enough love to go around. **Love is not a finite resource.**

We suggest that you reach out to other moms who are pregnant with multiples via online or local support groups for mothers of multiples (see **Resources**). These groups can be a source of companionship and also of practical information on everything from how to manage feedings to how to get your babies on the same sleep schedule. Though you don't have to plan for these specific challenges in your first trimester, learning that other mothers have solved what seem like impossible questions may be comforting.

Medically, a multiple pregnancy is considered a high-risk pregnancy. Carrying two or more babies is a greater physical demand. A multiples pregnancy means more tests, more doctors' visits, and a higher possibility of a C-section and other medical interventions when the babies are born. All of this medical attention may make you feel anxious, but it doesn't mean you're not well or that anything will go wrong for your babies. It may be helpful to reframe your thoughts this way: You and your medical team are prepared for the worst case but expecting the best.

What's your advice for single mothers during pregnancy?

Depending on your circumstances, facing pregnancy without a partner can feel scary, freeing, or somewhere in between. As you might expect, the emotional experiences of single motherhood is different depending on your circumstances. If you are a planned single mother by choice, if your partner passed away, if you've decided not to involve the father of the baby, if your partner hasn't wanted to be involved, or if you're separated, your stressors and joys may be different.

If you're feeling irritated by "couple envy," we encourage you to remember that every relationship has its challenges. As demanding as raising a child on your own is, it can be a blessing to be spared from having to share decision-making about parenting with someone who isn't a good partner to you or parent to your child.

That doesn't mean you aren't allowed to feel grief and anger. As one of our patients shared: "Sometimes at two a.m., when I'm alone, I feel really mad at her father. I had a dad who was there for me in all ways, and it's sad to realize that my daughter won't have that."

We encourage you to try not to let those feelings, alongside any disappointment, eclipse the gratitude you may be feeling about your pregnancy. As shared by one of our patients who planned a pregnancy as a single mother by choice: "After my mom died, I realized that even though I wasn't yet in a relationship, I didn't want to lose the opportunity to become a mom. I think I always knew more than anything that I wanted a child, and I didn't want to have to wait for a relationship to have that in my life. I'm a doer, and so getting pregnant was like checking something huge off my bucket list in a way that made me feel so alive, fulfilled, and in control of my life."

And just because you are not partnered in a traditional romantic way doesn't mean that you are alone. During pregnancy you can start building your support network to include all of the family and friends who can help you. One of our patients gave this advice: "You need your crew—that's what kept me from feeling alone. And it doesn't have to be huge. I decided to choose just one of my friends who was a mom to talk to as my go-to person for advice. I trusted her and her parenting style, and it was really helpful to not have too much input from different people."

Your circle of support may include longtime friends and family, and also the broader scope of new relationships from a local group of single mothers or an online virtual village. During pregnancy, it's going to be important to start thinking about how you'll negotiate child care and other financial and logistical arrangements. One of our patients said, "Having other friends who are single moms is key. I look around at my single-mom friends and think if they can do it, I can do it. We also babysit for each other—as a single mom, you need to still be able to have a social life."

As a single mom, you're going to have to be your own soul mate and your own co-parent. Imagine the environment you would want for your child and figure out how to create it on your own. One of our patients shared this strategy: "Know that it's possible to give your child an atmosphere of peace and calm even though you are alone. Having a child is often a way to learn about yourself. When you're alone and no one's watching, you sometimes feel like you could slip into bad behavior, so be your own partner and watch yourself. Another single mom told me that she pretends that there's a camera watching just to make sure she's as much of her best self as she can be with her kids." Please see our **Resources** for links to supportive communities and tools.

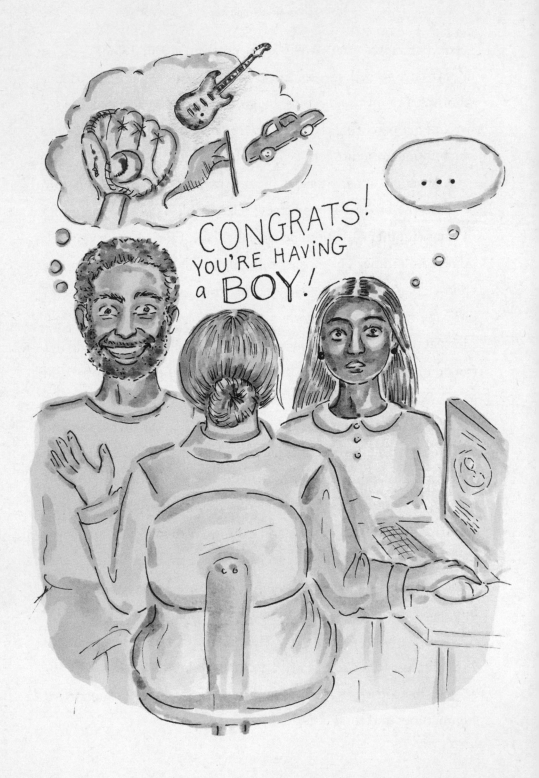

The Second Trimester

Fantasy vs. Reality

Some women hold off from getting excited about their pregnancy until the second trimester, when they can see the fetal anatomy more clearly on the ultrasound and hear from a doctor that the miscarriage risk is now very low. If you're generally cautious about getting close to new people until you're confident that the relationship is a "sure thing," your attachment to your pregnancy may deepen more slowly, as with someone wading into a pool one careful toe at a time. As one of our patients described it, "I had gone through a totally unexpected pregnancy loss before, and it hit me hard. This time, I waited until the second trimester to call her 'my baby.' In the first trimester, it just felt safer to say 'the pregnancy' until the odds were better that I wasn't going to have to deal with another loss."

As your bond with your baby deepens in the second trimester, you'll actually develop a connection with *two* babies: the one physically growing in your body and another that's alive in your imagination. We'll call this your fantasy baby, and she's just as important as the one you'll eventually hold in your arms. But it's helpful to remember that they're not the same.

All of us play out our greatest hopes, wishes, and fears like films in our heads, and many women started dreaming about motherhood when they were children. What did you think pregnancy would be like? How did you picture yourself as a mother? How did you imagine your child? Over the years, if you've struggled with infertility or finding a partner, or have otherwise chosen to delay getting pregnant, these fantasies may have become intensified by yearning.

Paying attention to your fantasies can teach you a lot about yourself. Your fantasies also reflect what you've gleaned from the experiences of your own mother and other female relatives. Do you have memories of your mother telling you that having children was her most meaningful and rewarding experience? Was there an aunt who warned you that having children caused her marriage to unravel, so watch out? All of that history finds its way into how you imagine yourself as a mother.

If you look closely, you'll see that the community and culture in which you live, books you've read, movies and media you've consumed have also shaped your imagination about motherhood. Maybe you've watched the same talk-show host on TV for over a decade—you've heard about her hands-on attention to her children, seen her career boom, and watched her body shrink back to model size after pregnancy. Maybe you've looked up to her as an ideal, hoping that you might be able to accomplish what she has with her cheerful and self-deprecating humor.

Or your fantasies may be a reaction against—rather than an imitation of—mothering you've seen. You may envision a future family that fills in the holes of what was missing before and transforms you into the person you've always wanted to be. You may imagine that having a child will make you feel more confident, as if you've finally accomplished something important to be proud of. You may imagine that cuddling with a baby will keep you calm and never feeling lonely. You may imagine that your baby will be so adorable that you and your partner will be too busy laughing to bicker. You may imagine that you'll be so busy and productive while caring for your child that you won't have any time to procrastinate on projects.

In psychology, we call this high-gloss vision of our future selves an "idealization," meaning a view of life that is "all good." Idealization carries the danger of unrealistic expectations for what real life will feel like, but it's not necessarily unhealthy if you can keep perspective that these thoughts are just hopeful daydreams. Idealized fantasies can be a fun way to emotionally prepare for your new role, and for many people, these all-happy daydreams are much more comfortable than waiting for an unknown future that will have both ups and downs.

Be curious about your daydreams or fantasies, but do your best not to judge or get too attached to them. **Fantasies sometimes tell us what we desire or fear, but they don't predict what will happen, what we actually need, or what will make us happy.** Think back to the fantasies you may have had about your future partner—they likely didn't predict exactly whom you ended up with, and hopefully that worked out just fine or even for the better. You can't map out intimate relationships in your head; you have to share experiences with people and see how they feel in real life. This is true in marriage as well as motherhood.

Remembering that hopeful fantasies are just that will also help you when your imagination lurks to darker scenarios. One of our patients told us, "When I think of a baby in my arms, I get nervous. What if I can't handle it? Will I really love my child? I hated babysitting as a teenager, and I still don't feel comfortable when I'm around my friends' kids. What if, every time I hear my baby cry, I want to run away?" These kinds of daydream-nightmares may be upsetting, but they can also be oddly soothing if they help you face your deepest fears through your imagination and leave you feeling more in control.

Try to think of your fantasies as questions rather than answers. They are a creative exploration of your own desires and concerns, and they are much more about you and your past than about your future relationship with your baby. Especially if your fantasies feel frightening, consider talking about them with your partner or someone else you trust. Describing your nightmares out loud can take away their power—you'll see how unlikely a worst-case scenario is, or how what seemed horrible when you imagined it can actually be a manageable problem.

By the time your "real" baby arrives, you'll have already developed feelings about your fantasy baby, and those feelings can be powerful enough that reality may disappoint you when it doesn't align with your vision. This often comes up around wanting a boy or a girl, as we've found that many pregnant women have vivid fantasies of their child's sex. Sure, everyone says they'll love their baby as long as it's healthy, but that's often because they feel ungrateful to admit that they have a secret wish for one or the other.

Many women fantasize about having a girl because they find it easier to picture her. Often they're replaying memories from their own childhood and imagining a little girl as a mini-me or a future best friend. A girl's body may also just be more familiar, easier to think about in terms of diaper changes and someday having The Talk. Some women may fantasize about going shopping with a daughter, if that's what they enjoy, and feel anxious when they try to imagine playing with a son because they "don't know how to do boy stuff" like roughhousing, if that's what they remember about their interactions with an older brother.

On the other hand, a woman may fantasize about having a little boy if she had an easy connection with a little brother, or if she had a competitive or difficult relationship with her sister or mother and doesn't want to repeat those dynamics in another female bond. If she views her husband as happy and unflappable, she may imagine a son with that personality rather than a daughter who might inherit some of her flaws.

Some women who fantasized about mothering a girl have told us that parenting a boy turned out to be easier in spite of their initial disappointment. There can be a number of reasons for this, but one may be that the more obvious the physical differences are, the easier it may be to remember that your child is a unique and separate person.

We encourage you to remember that biological sex is no guarantee of your child's interests and disposition. Your daughter may love sports and hate shopping; your son may be sensitive and great at talking about his feelings. (Biological sex is also no guarantee of gender or sexual orientation.) When your baby is first born, the anatomy will be all you know about him or her. But soon enough, you'll get to know your child's quirks and personality, related to gender and beyond. Whether the baby is the sex you wished for or not, he or she will be full of surprises.

Pink and Blue

By the second trimester, you'll be given some opportunities to find out the sex of your baby before arrival. There's no right answer on whether it's better to find out the sex or wait, so consider the question and talk about it with your partner, ideally before your doctor puts you on the spot to decide.

Here are some pros and cons of finding out your baby's sex early, to help you and your partner think through this decision:

Pros:

- You may feel more in control during the pregnancy because you know something tangible about your child—this may be calming.
- Finding out if it's a boy or a girl may make the baby feel more real, which might help you feel more emotionally attached.
- For some parents, this information helps to make choices around baby clothing or nursery design in advance.
- You have more time to decide on the baby's name if your decision is based on sex.
- If it's different than what you had hoped for, you have time to deal with feelings of disappointment.

Cons:

- If the news is disappointing, you'll have to sit with it for a while, whereas if you find out in the delivery room, you'll have plenty of other things to focus on—like having just given birth and the joy of meeting your healthy baby. One patient said, "I wanted to wait to find out at the birth because I knew that if it was a boy, I would love him because he was my baby. I knew I would feel that way once he was born, but might not feel that way during pregnancy—I would have more time to think about wanting a girl."

- You may experience stress if you decide not to tell others the sex and don't like keeping secrets.

- If you decide to tell people the sex, you'll have to deal with their reactions and feelings. One patient's mother-in-law said: "You're having another girl? Do you think you'll plan on having a third after this one so you can give your husband a son?"

- You'll miss out on a surprise that, for some parents, contributes to the magic of birth.

- Knowing the baby's sex can feed in to intense, detailed fantasies about what she will be like—which can be a problem if you're prone to getting too attached to an imagined future.

If you and your partner disagree about whether to find out in advance, we recommend sharing your personal feelings rather than getting into a debate about the abstract pros and cons. If you aren't able to come to a natural compromise, we usually advise letting the person with the more distressed, or intense, feelings "win." For example, if you think it will be fun to be surprised when you give birth, but your wife is anxious about unknowns and will feel calmer if she knows in advance, it may be worth soothing her fears by sacrificing your fun surprise. Consider what other decisions—such as you getting first dibs on picking a name—can help balance it out. In other words, pick your battles and decide if this one is more important to you than other things you and your partner will have to negotiate.

One of the central tasks of parenting is to see your children for who they are, not who you think they should be. **The more you can remember that your child's experience in the world is not the same as yours, the more empathic a parent you'll become.** You'll have the chance to work on this for years, but we recommend you start now, as you think about what you're hoping to get from your future child and mothering.

One patient of ours said, "I didn't have a great relationship with my mom growing up—she was really self-centered. I really wanted a girl so I could experience a better version of the mother/

daughter relationship." Her desire for a healing experience was totally understandable, but viewing her daughter's life as a canvas for repainting and repairing her own childhood may have become self-centered, too. Because she could identify this fantasy before her baby girl's arrival, she was able to do what her mom couldn't: reflect on her own emotional needs so that her parenting could be focused on her daughter's.

What's in a Name?

For most parents, choosing a child's name feels both exciting and daunting, as if you are writing the first page in the book of your child's life and the word choice is up to you.

If your family has specific expectations, the control may not feel entirely in your hands. Your relatives may nudge you with requests, since names are often viewed as meaningful leaves hanging on the family tree. Your mother may say that you owe it to your grandfather to carry on his name because he brought the family to America or paid for your education. Your father may say that it's only right to honor his sister's name because she never had children and helped to raise you. Your sister may say that not using your deceased mother's name would be an insult to her and a sign that you didn't love her. As with other experiences in your pregnancy, it's heavy to be handed this kind of baggage from your family members, who are experiencing your baby's life as a part of their larger history. There's no right answer for how to think about this, but one thing to consider is that there are other ways to show respect for your ancestors if you'd rather not do so through your child's name.

Friends and family may have judgmental feedback about your name choices. "A girl named Jordan won't be seen as feminine" or "Since you married a person from a different ethnicity, the least you could do to honor your heritage is to give your child a name from our culture." Remember that these reactions are ultimately about the person who expresses them, and if they're upsetting, do your best to brush them off. If it helps, you may be able to remember other, similar examples with this same intrusive person that seemed like a big drama at the time but ultimately faded, such as a request to include a tradition in your wedding ceremony.

As with other inappropriate behavior you may encounter, the way you deal with things publicly doesn't have to dictate your private decisions. You can say, "That gives me a lot to think about" without making any promises. This type of response can help you draw a boundary so that you can keep a line of privacy. It may seem obvious, but we strongly advise that you and your partner have a discussion ahead of time on how you will handle family feedback about names so you're both prepared and can support each other. If you're worried about judgmental feedback, consider not telling anyone your chosen name until the baby is born. It's much harder to respond to a named baby with criticism than when your plans are still up in the air.

Choosing a name can also be weighed with your own fantasies of whom you want your child to be, or a way to show how creative you plan to be as parents. **But remember, just as your child will announce her own personality, her identity will infuse her name, rather than vice versa.** If you're digging deep to find a name that will be unique or stylish, try to imagine what it's going to feel like for your child to live with that name for decades to come. A name that's very cute or exceptional may be a source of embarrassment if your child ends up in the clergy or a federal judge. A child's name should not be a burden.

And if you can't decide on a name right now? Relax. You can wait until the third trimester or even after your baby is born. Sometimes people are most creative when they're not focusing on a specific problem. If you take the pressure off yourself, inspiration may come to you when you least expect it.

Changing Shape

We've found that the second trimester is when many of our patients start talking about weight-related anxiety. Weight gain is usually seen as a negative in our culture, especially for women, who are often raised to think that the ideal body is small and slim. So, whether you're gaining weight all over or just in your belly, the physical changes of pregnancy can be emotionally challenging. One of our patients told us, "In the second trimester, I'd started to show, but I hadn't really 'popped.' I was worried people would think I was just gaining weight, so I did things like rubbing my belly or arching my back so they'd see I was pregnant."

On the other hand, some women love their new curves. One of

our patients said, "This was finally a change from the same body I've had my whole life—thin, athletic, flat-chested—so I loved having boobs and feeling round and feminine for the first time ever." Another patient told us, "I'd always been self-conscious about my body, growing up as a chubby kid. Being pregnant let me enjoy having a bigger body without worrying about all the shame. I started wearing form-fitting clothing I never would've considered before. I was getting bigger because I had a baby inside me, and that felt awesome."

One of the reasons we love the word "matrescence" is that it sounds like "adolescence," and being pregnant is like going through puberty all over again. Your body is sprouting new curves; your hair may get thick and lustrous, or it may get flat and weird. Your hormones go nuts, and it shows. A pimple erupts smack in the center of your forehead like a nasty third eye, and the faded preteen stretch marks hugging your hips spread anew like purple vines creeping toward your protruding middle.

By now, your adolescence was probably a decade or two ago (or longer), and you've had the chance to grow into your appearance and figure out your look from head to toe. While you may still be struggling to embrace your body before pregnancy, you've hopefully found a routine for feeling secure. In pregnancy, your whole system can be thrown off. As your appearance transforms, you may catch your unfamiliar reflection in the bathroom mirror and think, *I don't recognize myself.* This is a major component of the identity shift of matrescence—your body stops feeling like the body you've known, and that's even before taking into account the challenging feelings that can come with gaining weight.

If you've spent most of your life monitoring your weight, your changing shape may make you feel like you're losing control of yourself. Sadly, for some women, pregnancy is the first time in their adult life when they're not actively trying to lose weight. This can be a chance to heal a fraught relationship with your body. If the process of weighing in at every prenatal visit is troubling you, you can stand on the scale with your back to the display and just ask your practitioner to tell you whether or not you're gaining at a healthy rate, without giving you the exact number.

If you have struggled with an eating disorder in the past, it's important that you discuss it with your provider (and see **Resources**). Even if it's painful or embarrassing to talk about your relationship to food and your body, your health and your baby's depend on it, because eating enough calories is essential for growing a healthy baby. If your doctor thinks that you're not gaining enough weight, and there's no medical reason for this deficit, you might reflect on whether there's an emotional origin. The same goes for overeating— if your doctor is concerned that you're gaining more weight than is healthy (and there isn't a medical reason), it may be worth asking yourself if you're eating beyond hunger to soothe other feelings, or having a reaction to the freedom of eating for two that is morphing from liberated to self-destructive. Either way, consulting with a nutritionist or therapist might be a good idea.

While it can be challenging to disconnect weight loss from

your metric of healthy eating, it can also be an amazing learning experience: What does healthy eating look like for you when it's not just about eating *less*? Many of our patients have told us that learning how to "eat for the baby" is easier than making healthy choices for their own bodies.

 Eating for Mental Health

While many books have been written about nutrition and pregnancy, as psychiatrists we do offer our patients some basic advice for healthy eating that also supports mental health:

- **Eat fresh, whole foods.** Focusing on unprocessed foods will help to avoid added chemicals and benefit from the freshest produce, healthy proteins, healthy fats, and whole grains.

- **Eat colorfully.** The more colorful the foods are on your plate, the more nutrient-rich they probably are. Think orange sweet potatoes, red beets, blue blueberries, and green kale.

- **Healthy choices.** Focus on what to eat rather than what to avoid. Focus on the positive ways you want to nurture yourself, rather than negative thoughts about deprivation. For example: "I will eat three servings of vegetables" instead of "No candy." Sometimes, when people feel deprived by restrictions, they end up binging rather than benefitting from moderation.

- **Don't fear fat.** Fats are the building blocks of your brain's gray matter (home base for the brain chemicals that involve anxiety and depression) and of your baby's growing brain. Moderate amounts of fat from grass-fed meat, full-fat dairy, eggs, omega-3 fatty fish like salmon, nuts, avocado, and oils like olive oil are good for your brain and your baby's brain development.

Pregnancy, like puberty, is freaky. But growing a baby is also a gorgeous, powerful, creative act. You may feel like a mess, but try to think of yourself as a work of art. As one of our patients said, "I could pretend I've transcended body image concerns, but that's simply not true and virtually impossible in our society. Perhaps I could have exercised more or eaten a little healthier, but I've also listened to my body and allowed for the cravings it's desired—likely for the first time ever. Instead of staring into the mirror, thinking, *Ugh, how did my face get so fat,* I'm going to do my best to say: *I'm making a human with the love of my life. That's why I look different right now, and there's nothing more beautiful in the world than that.*" (Or some other mantra that feels right to you.)

Screening

In your second trimester, your practitioner will talk to you about medical screening and, in particular, whether or not testing, like amniocentesis, is recommended. Which tests are necessary and which are optional are complicated questions. Some invasive tests can help you make decisions about termination or medical intervention early, but the procedures may also carry some risk.

Your provider may make suggestions about recommended tests but not tell you what you should do. **This may be the first time in your life when a doctor has left a medical decision in your hands, and for many people, that feels stressful.** "Isn't my doctor the expert?" they ask. "Why is this my decision?" Your doctor can't guarantee that an invasive procedure won't disrupt a pregnancy; it's up to you to decide whether to take that risk. She can't tell you whether you should continue with a pregnancy if a test indicates a problem.

Your decision to test or not may be informed by your and your partner's religion, culture, family, and values. Your doctor can help you weigh the risks and benefits of testing, but the final decision is yours and your partner's. You might want to test for the reassurance of good news. You might forgo testing if you wouldn't terminate a pregnancy under any circumstances. Even if you wouldn't terminate a pregnancy, you might want to have all the medical information testing might yield to prepare, so you can have your emotional and medical support systems in place.

This may be the first of many decisions that you will make

about the health and well-being of your child where there is no obvious "right answer" or instruction manual. Down the road, your pediatrician may offer advice but leave decisions about circumcision, sleep training, weaning, and potty training up to you, so it's helpful to get oriented to this experience and try trusting yourself as the grown-up who knows what's best for your child. Building this confidence isn't easy, as one patient described: "When my doctor turns to me and asks me these serious questions, I sometimes imagine I'm on one of those prank reality TV shows—my parents are going to show up and say, *Just kidding, of course we'd never trust you, a person who sleeps through her alarm and runs out of toilet paper, to be in charge of a baby!*" Over time you'll learn that much of parenthood sometimes requires a fake-it-till-you-make-it strategy; you might just have to give your best performance of what a wise adult would do, even if you still feel like a scared kid inside.

If you're thirty-five or older, your doctor may refer to your "advanced maternal age" as a reason for additional testing. This isn't a personal criticism but the technical term for your age bracket. A woman who gives birth after the age of thirty-five has a higher risk of some medical complications, including certain chromosomal changes that could cause genetic conditions for the fetus, so it's a benchmark for increased clinical vigilance and medical monitoring. But this awkward language leaves some women feeling insecure or judged.

We wish that doctors could find a better term to explain the helpful extra layer of care to women, as "advanced maternal age"

sounds like they're about to send you to a retirement home. But this insensitive language may be preparation for any less than ideal bedside manner you may unfortunately experience with health care professionals. For example, during an ultrasound, a technician might say audibly, "Wow, small for sixteen weeks" or announce, "I have to call the doctor now," and not explain why before she rushes out, leaving you waiting for thirty minutes of torture until the doctor arrives.

Every time you're wearing a paper gown and talking to someone who is fully clothed or wearing a white coat, every time you're putting your feet in stirrups or having a conversation about your health, body, and baby, you're probably going to feel more exposed than the health care worker on the other side of the conversation. But even though being a patient may make you feel vulnerable, you are always allowed to speak up and give direct feedback to any health professional who is being insensitive. For most of us, putting our feelings into words is an important part of feeling safe, and more in control, when we're at our most helpless. You have our permission to give polite feedback like "It was very stressful to be left hanging and have to wait so long for that information." Or "I'd rather not have this discussion until I can put my clothes on." Or "I need to talk to my partner before making that decision." Or "Yes, I used a donor egg. Do you have to mention it at every appointment?"

Whatever screenings you choose, it's normal to be antsy, sleepless, or irritable before the test and as you wait for the results. Many women tell us they can't concentrate at work or enjoy socializing as

they wait out those few uncertain days. Many women are afraid the test will be painful or will hurt their baby, though odds are low for both. Even if you know that the chance you'll hear upsetting news is very unlikely, it's hard to not focus on that possibility as you wait for the doctor's phone call.

Managing Anxiety While Waiting for Medical Results

If you're feeling anxious while waiting for test results, we suggest that you put your rational mind in the driver's seat. A psychological term for being able to integrate your logic with your emotions is called using your "wise mind."

Try this writing exercise:

- Write down a few affirming sentences to use as mantras. For example: *I'll get the news soon and then the discomfort of waiting will be over.*

- Write down the reasons you decided to have the test, reminding yourself that no matter what the outcome is, getting tested was the right decision for you. If it helps you feel more in control, you may consider writing down a plan for whom you will seek

advice from if you have to deal with any complicated and upsetting medical information.

- If you feel too uncomfortable sitting and waiting and you feel the need to "do something," try an activity that would be comforting, like listening to music, or distracting, like organizing your closet.

- If you decided not to have any diagnostic tests, you may also have moments of doubt. If you're worrying about this decision, write down the reasons you're not doing the test, then read this list to put your rational mind in charge when you're feeling anxious.

Facing the Choice of Termination

If you receive difficult news from the results of testing or an anatomy scan, you may be faced with the decision of whether or not to continue the pregnancy. Figuring out what you need to do is a painful and personal process that will involve educating yourself about the medical situation, speaking to genetic or other counselors, and soul-searching on your own and with your partner.

For some couples, the decision, however heart-wrenching, is obvious. Others end up realizing that what feels personally right for their situation is out of line with their political or religious beliefs. If you're surprised with how your partner reacts, remember, this is an unexpected loss for him or her, too. No matter how close you are, you may have different responses to trauma based on your past histories. If you've learned that keeping busy and talking about distracting topics helps you stay calm when you're upset, you may find it hard if your partner can't get off the couch or talk about anything else. If your different needs are pushing you apart during this time when you need each other's support, a mental health professional or counselor can help you understand your different reactions.

One of our patients was told that her baby wasn't growing due to a medical condition, and she had to deal with her mother's incorrect opinion that the problem could have been prevented if she had eaten more. If you anticipate that your family's reaction will make the experience more difficult, then you may want to wait until you've gotten through the most upsetting stages to tell them. If they continue to want to talk about how well the pregnancy is going before you're ready to tell them about your medical complications, there is nothing wrong with avoiding their calls for a few days and telling them you're not up to talking or not feeling well. If you feel guilty, remind yourself that this is your body and it's okay to keep private boundaries until you feel ready to talk.

Many mothers who have to make a choice about medical termination tell us that they are left feeling guilty that their body somehow failed their baby or that they're doing the "wrong thing." If you're beating yourself up about your decision, try to remember that this situation, whatever the outcome, was caused by a biological event and not anything you did wrong. You may be angry at yourself, your doctor, and the universe before you are able to accept what is happening. That's a natural part of grieving a loss.

Allow yourself to process this news in any way that feels right to you. Some women may send a group email to let friends know, or ask family to explain. Others may lock the door and turn off the phone until they're ready to face the world. If you don't want to see friends or family right away, don't. They'll be there to comfort you when you're ready.

It can be excruciating to return to work and your usual routines if you have to tell people over and over that you're no longer pregnant. It may be helpful to rehearse how you want to let people know and what to say that will make you feel the most comfortable under such upsetting circumstances. We suggest something direct that makes your needs clear: "I lost the pregnancy. I don't want to talk about the details. Thank you for asking." Or "I lost the baby. I'm really sad, but I'm hanging in. Thank you for asking." You may be the kind of person who is supersensitive to making others feel comfortable, but even if they want to hear about your pregnancy loss, that doesn't mean that you have to talk about it. You've just suffered a loss and need to focus on how to get through one day at a time.

One of our patients said, "We lost the baby, and I was recovering from the procedure. My husband's birthday party had been scheduled for a few weeks after, and I was dreading facing all our friends. I would have never suggested we cancel his party, because that would have made me feel like a failure as a wife in addition to a mother, but he offered to reschedule it. Nothing like this had happened to any of my friends—I felt so sad and weak and angry at the same time. I just wasn't ready to see them yet." Later, this patient told us that when she finally was able to face her friends, several of them shared that they, too, had experienced miscarriages (but, like her, hadn't felt comfortable speaking about their experiences of loss in the open).

The Secret's Out

Telling Your Social Circle

In the second trimester, when you announce your pregnancy to your larger circle of friends, many will hug you with happiness, and some may even squeal or jump up and down, as you'd expect. But the ones who have always been a little high-maintenance (think back to your wedding, their wedding, or other milestones, and you'll know whom we mean) may, as usual, make things more complicated. In their defense, because your peers are also in their reproductive years, many of them (the delicate as well as the more thick-skinned ones) may simultaneously be going through their own demanding conception, pregnancy, and parenting experiences. Their reactions to your pregnancy may range from slightly strained to wildly inappropriate if they are wrestling with their own uncomfortable feelings. Even your friends who do not have children may have strong reactions as they relate to your plan for a vision of life that will diverge from theirs.

Depending on your relationship, you may feel that you can be honest about your hurt feelings if you feel like a friend is letting you down. More often, you may have to simply accept that not everyone will be able to—or want to—share your excitement.

Some of your friends may react with an edge of competition. We're not excusing any bad behavior, but it might help you understand if you put yourself in their shoes. When your single friend says, "Well, I guess I'll stop inviting you to girls' night out," she might unintentionally be excluding you because she anticipates feeling rejected down the road when you pass on late nights to stay home and rest. When one of our patients told her friend that she was pregnant, her friend said, "Wow, everything just falls into place for you—you've been trying, what, five minutes?" In fact, it had been almost a year. When our patient asked her friend why she was being so flip and ungenerous about her pregnancy news, she learned that the friend had been struggling with fertility treatments and was feeling like everyone else had it easier.

We've heard women who have had miscarriages say that seeing a pregnant woman or attending a baby shower can make them so jealous and frustrated that their reaction borders on rage. They may feel ashamed that they can't be happy for you, and may distance themselves from you. As one patient of ours described: "My best friend from childhood and I were pregnant together, and then she had a miscarriage. It was this giant elephant in our relationship— she wouldn't ask me about my pregnancy, and I was scared to ask her how she was feeling. Instead of mourning her baby while celebrating mine, we ended up doing neither, which just felt sad and empty."

If you have a friend who you know may be struggling with her own fertility-related hurt, it might be better to tell her about your pregnancy in a private conversation rather than in a group. Think about the language you use. Just one empathic comment, like "I know you also want to be a mother, and I hope one day I can be there for your good news," is all it takes to let this friend know you're thinking about her. That being said, if you feel like you don't have the bandwidth to deal with your more sensitive friends, you can tell them in an email or some other way that gives you both distance to protect yourselves (and your friendship) from the most painful early reactions.

One of our patients shared this advice: "I was going to visit my best friend who lived far away for her birthday. She had been through a divorce and a recent diagnosis of a chronic illness, so she wasn't getting pregnant anytime soon. I knew that if I sprung my pregnancy news on her in person, it might take over the whole weekend, which was supposed to be fun and about her. Even though it was less personal, I called her to tell her before the trip. She was quiet over the phone, but later told me it was helpful to give her a heads-up because she had some time to deal with her own mixed feelings first." Even though telling a close friend over phone, text, or email can feel less intimate, for some it's the more thoughtful approach because it gives them a little more space and time if you suspect they may have conflicted feelings.

While many women are eager to make pregnancy announcements on social media, we encourage you to think before you post. Once something is posted, you won't be able to control who knows about your pregnancy and when they know. This is particularly important if you haven't told far-flung relatives or your boss or colleagues yet. And you should think about how you would feel in a worst-case scenario if you had a medical complication and then had to answer people's questions about your pregnancy online.

Consider also how you may be influenced by the social media culture that encourages women to boast about their pregnancies and children. Are you posting so that the people who love you can share in your happiness? Or are you manufacturing an artificial, idealized moment?

Remember that what you say and how you say it matters. One of our patients who had a prior miscarriage tearfully told us that one of her friends announced her pregnancy on Facebook. The caption? "Now I'm in the Mommy Club!" Of course she was happy for her friend, but it was a club from which she was excluded. We're not saying a new mother shouldn't spread the news and celebrate, but try to consider if you're contributing to the social media culture that treats motherhood like just another step up in social status.

Telling at Work

Many women wait as long as they can to announce their pregnancy at work. Because your coworkers and community may respond with their own questions about your maternity leave, it may make sense to put off this delivery of the news until you've passed through the higher-risk window of the first trimester or screening tests. Waiting to tell can give you the feeling of being more in control by helping you direct the flow of information. Or it can be stressful if you're worried about people suspecting or how people will react to your having kept "a secret."

How smoothly the process goes will depend in part on how you handle it, and in part on your workplace culture. In a perfect world, you'll have a paid maternity leave and coworkers who have already had good experiences using it and returning. But if you don't have positive models to follow, you may worry about how your coworkers and boss will react. Some women fear that they will be taken less seriously professionally. Some feel guilty, as if they're asking for special treatment or dumping their colleagues with extra work just because they're taking a maternity leave. Some women are afraid that their employer will subtly (or not so subtly) look for ways to sideline them.

Most women spend a lot of time thinking about how to tell a boss about their pregnancy. But there may be other people, like your assistant (if you have one) or direct report, cubicle mate, or others who may guess or need to know earlier. The benefits of telling a person like this before your boss is that he may be able to cover for you if you have to leave for an appointment or are not feeling well. However, this comes with the risk that your boss could hear about it through office gossip before she hears it from you. One of our patients struggled with this: "It was hard at work because one of my coworkers had already told my boss before I could. I don't think she was being malicious about it, just gossipy. But it threw me for such a loop because I went into the conversation not knowing that my boss already knew I was pregnant. I felt totally blindsided."

Before sitting down with your boss, review your company's maternity leave policy, and think about how it would apply to you. We suggest that you plan to take the full amount of leave permitted, and unless you're 100 percent sure you're not coming back, tell your boss you'll be returning to your job. **It's easier to come back to work early or decide not to return than to request an extension of your leave or ask for your job back later on.** Even if you've taken maternity leave before and think you know exactly how you'll feel, you may not be able to predict the experience of number two or three.

If you're feeling guilty about keeping your options open while telling your boss that you're sure to return, think about other situations when you might keep information about your future private from your boss—like if you were looking for a new job or received an offer from a competing company. Even better, imagine what a male executive would do: Would he sit down with his boss to talk about the job interviews he's been going on? No way! It is not expected that you tell your current employer when you're considering a new job until you're 100 percent sure that you're leaving—why should it be any different for plans post–maternity leave?

Our culture tells women they should feel guilty if they aren't compassionate caretakers. But in the workplace, especially if yours doesn't offer postpartum benefits that are the norm in other countries, we encourage you to put your needs first, and maybe even before your boss's (and yes, this applies to you even if you are the boss!).

Be professional and plan for your meeting with your boss. Even if you know her well, you may be pleasantly (or disturbingly) surprised by her reaction. If you're coming to her before telling the rest of the office, let her know. Especially if you anticipate that that public discussion about pregnancy will distract you from your work, you can ask her not to share the news or confirm any rumors until you are ready.

 Tips for Telling Your Boss

The following are some tips that may help when talking with your boss about your pregnancy:

- **Come prepared and know what you want to ask.** Research your company's policies by asking human resources. What's the policy on part-time? Working from home? Extra weeks off if you have a medical complication? Extra weeks you can add of unpaid time?
- **Don't have this conversation on the fly.** Schedule the meeting for a quiet part of the day.
- **Be empathic.** A statement like "I understand this news may

create a challenge for you and the company" makes it clear that you understand your leave will impact others. You're not apologizing for what you need, you're simply being thoughtful. This may go a long way, especially when you're asking for help.

- **Take work off her plate.** Offer suggestions about who should take on your work tasks/roles, and assure her that you will leave a clean desk and detailed instructions before you go.

- **Give yourself some wiggle room.** It is perfectly acceptable to say, "I don't have all my answers yet."

- **Protect yourself.** If your boss does become angry, try to deal with the behavior professionally and respectfully. Staying calm in the heat of the moment will give you time and clarity to figure out how best to respond. If you have any concerns that your boss may try to dock your pay or look for ways to fire you without cause, speak to your HR department. You can also find excellent legal advice from advocacy communities (see **Resources**).

Does telling your boss mean that you have to tell all your coworkers at the same time? Of course not. But you should consider getting ahead of the news before your bump asserts itself. Commenting on someone's body is generally not okay at work, but unfortunately, even in the workplace, a sense of appropriate boundaries can get blurry around pregnancy. Your coworkers probably wouldn't point out if you had a bad haircut, would they? But it's better to prepare for intrusive observations about your pregnancy so you know how to handle the situation before it arises. If someone asks whether you're pregnant and you're not ready to share the news, be polite but firm. You could say, "That's a very personal question." Or if you know the person well, try to deflect the question with humor: "Are you telling me I should be hitting the gym more?"

Many women feel guilty announcing their maternity leave to their team because they worry about burdening others. But making everyone happy all the time is an impossible expectation in most jobs, and in life. **Remember that pregnancy is a normal life event, not something you're doing to inconvenience your professional community.** If you have benefits, the expense of a possible medical leave has perhaps already been factored in to your and every employee's salary from the start. This should be a routine and regular entitlement of employment (one that isn't questioned in many other countries, where the benefits are universal and often more supportive than in the United States).

Change is always stressful for individuals and organizations, especially when it requires adjusting schedules and workflow. Your maternity leave means that others may have to take on additional work. Maybe you've heard your coworkers grumble about others taking maternity or medical leave, or your boss unravels when faced with unexpected staff changes. You may fear that people will be judging you behind your back. They may. But remember that their reaction is often about their own experiences and issues, not about you.

You can set the tone of your conversation with coworkers by remaining positive but professional and brief. Don't apologize! You've covered for colleagues when they were ill or on vacation, and you'll do so again when you return.

If you end up delivering or going on leave early, it may be the first time in your career that you have left work unfinished. Trust in yourself and others by letting them take over and accepting that the circumstances are out of your control. This can be demoralizing if your self-image and self-esteem are tied up in hearing the validation that you are a leader at work whom others can depend on and not vice versa. As humans, we all have times when we need to ask for help. If that's hard for you, there's no better time to practice getting comfortable with your discomfort than at the precipice of motherhood, because there will be many more times in the postpartum and beyond when you'll have to lean on others.

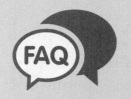 The following are some of the questions we hear most from our patients in the second trimester.

If I can't exercise during pregnancy, what else can I do to feel better?

Exercise has numerous benefits in pregnancy, including boosting mood and mitigating depression. But for some women, medical concerns or extreme tiredness make exercise a challenge.

If you have to take a break from your usual workout routines, the second trimester is a good time to establish new low-intensity habits to care for yourself physically and psychologically. Restorative activities like gentle yoga, stretching, and walking are good for your body and help to modulate stress hormones. This benefits both you and the baby, from reducing your blood pressure to helping prevent postpartum depression. It may even impact the development of the baby's nervous system and response to stress.

Consider other ways to connect to your body through mindfulness activities and experiences that engage all of your senses—sight, hearing, smell, taste, and touch. Unlike the cognitive techniques that use writing and logic to help reduce anxiety, mindfulness tools help redirect your attention from your thoughts to your physical sensations. When you're focused on your body's experience, you're forced to be present in the here and now—this helps to get you out of your head. Mindfulness shifts your attention away from your worries, and it has the additional benefit of harnessing your body's natural ability to soothe your nervous system.

Meditation, acupuncture, and prenatal massage can help. Deep breathing is one of the most simple and effective mindfulness approaches to try during pregnancy. For extra benefits, try constricting the back of your throat as you exhale. (If you do yoga, you know this as ujjayi breath. If you don't do yoga, aim for a Darth Vader sound.) This kind of breathing may stimulate the vagus nerve and act as a natural tranquilizer, releasing chemicals that signal your heart rate to slow and your whole nervous system to relax.

Try this: Breathe in through your nose to a count of four. Exhale completely through your mouth to a count of eight. Repeat four times. Deep breathing gets more challenging in the third trimester as your uterus expands to push up your diaphragm and compress your lung tissue, so start practicing now, and you'll be skilled to use this relaxation tool during labor and in the postpartum. For more practice, see **Resources**.

Other mindfulness approaches like sharing a meal with people who make you feel supported engages many senses and helps with the stress relief that comes from connecting to community. Listening to calming music may lower your blood pressure before a doctor's appointment. If you can't go for a run in the park, you can still sit on the grass and enjoy being in nature—spending time outdoors may help you relax, improve memory, and stimulate the production of vitamin D.

And we may be among the first doctors to tell you that watching TV is another acceptable way to lower your levels of stress. Zoning out when you have a lot on your mind can quiet rumination and help you reengage with feelings of pleasure, especially if the effort of socializing feels like more than you can handle right now.

Anything you can do that helps you feel centered can help lower your body's stress response. All these, and sex, of course, are healthy ways to support your mind/body wellness from the outside in.

What do I need to know about pregnancy sex?

At different times in your pregnancy, you may experience a range of feelings about sex: very horny, wanting space, gross, cuddly but anxious about penetration, like you want to have sex but only in pitch-black darkness so you don't have to look at your body, or a confusing combination of all of the above. Every woman has a slightly different sexual response to her hormonal fluctuations and the physical changes of pregnancy.

Your body and chemistry are changing by the day, and no matter how empathic your partner might be, his body and chemistry aren't. If your partner is wanting sex but you're feeling off, try to explain what's going on with your libido so she knows it's about your body and not a rejection of her. Yes, these types of conversations are scary. But ignoring your changing sex life can create distance and tension in your relationship, especially if having sex is the way that you normally stay connected.

You might be psychologically blocked from wanting sex if you can't get thoughts of the baby out of your head. Your body used to be all yours. Now there are literally three of you in bed together. If you've been getting used to being naked and spreading your legs for checkups, you may have started to feel like your genitals are more for function than recreation. Maybe you're upset about the weight you've gained; maybe you've stopped grooming your pubic hair or started wearing underwear that is more practical than pretty. It's normal to feel confused about your new physical experience as both a mother and a lover. Think about what parts of your pre-pregnancy sexual identity you can stay connected to, or how you might find a new sexuality that has space for your changing body and behaviors.

Your partner may be aroused by your extra curves or the fertility-goddess arc of your belly. Go with it! Pregnancy sex is a different experience, and you should try it. It can bring you and your partner closer as you explore your new body and help him to appreciate what's going on with you. You can ask your provider any physical questions, such as what positions would be most comfortable.

However, some partners find pregnancy itself to be a turnoff. If your partner has put you on the "mother" pedestal, he may see you as pure or saintly, maybe even associating to his own mother, and may no longer want to devour you. If this is happening, try to be patient with him and give him time to consider that just because you're about to take on the role of matriarch of the family doesn't mean you're no longer a sexual being.

If your partner tells you she's not attracted to your changing shape, this will be painful to hear. If your feelings are hurt, we encourage you to say so. Especially if you decided to get pregnant together, she doesn't have the right to be unkind, because you're the one making adjustments while carrying the baby for both of you.

Your partner may be scared, consciously or unconsciously, that the baby is aware when you're making love. Do your best to reassure her (and yourself) that your baby will not know that you're having sex—she's surrounded by a fluid-filled amniotic sac, protected by your uterine muscles. The baby cannot be touched by vaginal penetration because she is protected behind your closed cervix (which is the deepest part of your body accessible during vaginal penetration). All this means that it's not physically possible for a penis or fingers to bump into the baby. The rocking movements of sex may not feel any different to your baby than prenatal yoga or other physical activities.

Touching is an important aspect of bonding but doesn't have to be explicitly sexual. Cuddling while watching a movie or giving each other massages may help you feel connected in the way sex used to, or it may rekindle the sexual connection that is faltering. And if problems in your sex life are leading to fighting, you might want to consider meeting with a couples therapist to address these issues before they lead to growing distance or resentment.

When is the best time to move to a new home?

If your current home isn't the right place to raise a family, the second trimester can seem like the right time to move—you're more secure in the pregnancy than you were in the first trimester, but you're not too close to giving birth to consider taking on this big project. Moving, like new parenthood, is high on the list of life's most demanding events because it involves so much change. The first question you need to ask yourselves is: Do we want to move now, or would it be better to stay in our present home, at least for another year, so we don't have to deal with two transitions at one time?

Other topics for you and your partner to discuss: Can we afford to move? Do we want to move to be closer to parents, and if so, whose family "wins"? Do we need to consider a move to a less expensive community for cost or comfort—and how do we feel about this lifestyle adjustment or additional commute? How much space do we need to keep from wanting to kill each other when we're both sleep-deprived and our infant is screaming? If one of us is giving up a TV room or office to turn into the baby room, how will we negotiate this loss in privacy?

If all this feels too overwhelming, remember that you'll probably be fine staying where you are for now. From a practical point of view, you'll need only a small area for the baby's sleeping and diaper changing, and a comfortable spot to sit for feeding. A separate room to furnish for your baby's nursery might make you feel good, but in her first year, your baby will not know the difference.

Is it important for your relationship to take a "babymoon"?

Some couples like to take a trip during the second trimester, before they're medically advised to stay local in case of an early delivery in the third. We think this is a lovely idea, but not everyone wants, or is able, to spend the time or money. And some women find the prospect of traveling away from their doctors the opposite of relaxing.

This doesn't mean you can't take time before the baby arrives to reconnect and strengthen your bond with your spouse or partner. If you're not going to travel, think about the special little rituals that you enjoy as a couple. Maybe it's going out to a movie or concert, which will be harder to schedule when you need a babysitter. Maybe it's telling everyone you're out of town, while hiding at home and making out.

A babymoon, like a honeymoon, is about establishing physical and emotional intimacy, two things that often go by the wayside in the last weeks of pregnancy and the first months after a new baby comes home. But you don't need to fly to a tropical island to ensure that your relationship stays strong.

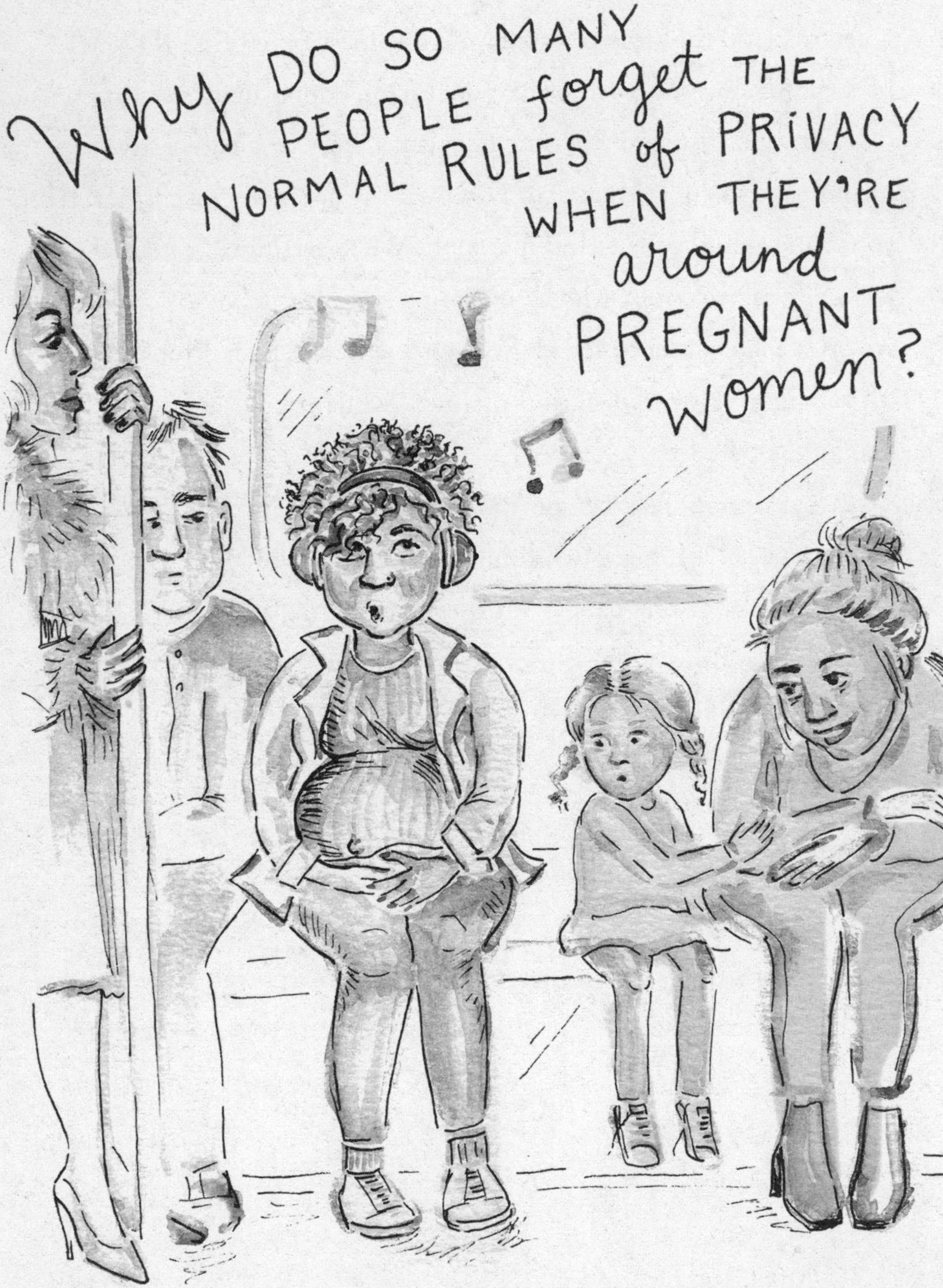
Why DO SO MANY PEOPLE forget THE NORMAL RULES of PRIVACY WHEN THEY'RE around PREGNANT women?

The Third Trimester

The End of an Era

The third trimester begins the home stretch of pregnancy and signals the impending end of your childless life. Part of you may want it to pass as quickly as possible so that you can meet your baby—and just get some physical relief. But another part of you may want to slow things down and linger a bit longer in your pre-baby life. **As excited as you are to become a mother, it may be scary when you stop and think about how life as you know it is about to end.** Up until now, you've existed in an adult world with an identity that's organized around yourself and, likely, other adults and adult commitments. Soon all this will change—with a special intensity if you're the primary caretaker.

Once the baby arrives, every role that contributes to your identity will feel transformed. Partner, spouse, lover, daughter, sister, friend, professional, colleague, pet owner, salsa dancer, college football tailgater, volunteer, activist—all the activities and relationships that make you feel like *you* will suddenly be different, both because of your new obligations and because of your new identity: mother.

Your family vacations will now have to be child-friendly. A pedicure with your sister will have to be around the baby's sleep schedule, or may not be affordable with your new budget. A spontaneous Sunday-afternoon movie with your girlfriends? Not going to happen unless it's On Demand, so you can feed your baby on demand, too. It might sound frivolous to be sad that you won't be able to wake up whenever you want and start your day scrolling through Instagram with your cup of coffee, but psychologically, it's not. When you're used to being able to do mostly what you want, when you want, and how you want, the changes of pregnancy and parenthood can make you feel like you're losing a part of yourself.

Identity Transitions and DIY Interpersonal Therapy (IPT)

In psychology, we call a life change that causes an intense shift in your identity and interpersonal relationships a "role transition." Psychology has zoomed in on these taxing transitions because they are high-stress times that, if ignored, can trigger depression and other kinds of psychological tension. This, as well as shifting hormones, may explain why the third trimester is a common time for postpartum depression to begin. (Yes, it frequently begins *during* pregnancy—more on that, and the difference between identity transitions and postpartum depression, in the **Appendix**.)

It's good to remind yourself that no matter how much you wanted and planned for motherhood, all of this identity shifting may leave you feeling out of control and disoriented at times. This is part of matrescence. But those negative feelings, and their impact on your mental well-being, can be mitigated. One way to do this is through interpersonal therapy (IPT), a psychological treatment designed to help people adjust to role transitions. IPT helps you regain your bearings so that the changes feel less overwhelming. It was developed for people struggling with depression, but we think it is a useful tool for any new mother.

We use IPT with many of our patients; its most helpful for the moments when you're feeling sad or frustrated by how your pregnancy or new life as a mother is requiring you to change. You can try out the main techniques on your own. And if this type of self-help doesn't make you feel better, we recommend talking about how you've been feeling with your doctor, who may refer you to a therapist who could professionally guide you through IPT or help in some other way.

Interpersonal Therapy (IPT)

IPT gives you a structured framework that involves four steps:

1. **Name what's upsetting you.** Sometimes we feel stressed without even knowing why. If your frustration and sadness feel amorphous, it may help to talk things through with your partner or a friend. Sometimes a friend who has been pregnant can relate from experience; other times it's simply the person who knows you best and will be best able to remind you of periods in your life when you've felt upset in a similar way. If you'd prefer privacy, journaling about how you're feeling may also be helpful—sometimes when we're writing, our self-awareness opens up if we can allow our minds to wander a bit.

2. **Articulate the identity change.** Now that you've named your sources of stress, think about how they are a disruption to your identity. Is this situation causing you to feel like you're losing part of who you are? Even seemingly trivial frustrations can connect to deep symbols of self. Recognizing that depth and putting it into words can help you better understand why the situation is challenging you in a way that feels core to who you are.

3. **Acknowledge your distress and take the time you need to accept your feelings.** Bad feelings don't exist only to be fixed— they can also provide signals about what's happening in our lives. Beyond that, not all negative feelings can be resolved. It's important to recognize your feelings, no matter how trivial or unhelpful they may seem, so that you can start thinking about how to work through them. You can cry it out, do yoga or meditate, punch a pillow, or "yell" about it into the ear of an understanding friend or family member until you're ready to accept what you cannot change and do your best to let go of your frustration.

4. **Come up with a plan for how to adapt to your new circumstances.** Once you identify the role change that's at the root of what's upsetting you, you can work to find a resolution. You can't go back to exactly who you were, but you can look for a way forward that adapts your values and priorities to your new situation and new identity. Think of this plan as narrative therapy: You're writing a new chapter for the story of your new identity.

Here's how one of our patients used an IPT-style approach to adapt to the lifestyle changes brought on by her pregnancy: "I'm happiest when I'm out and about. For as long as I can remember, I've spent Saturdays running errands and visiting friends. I spend hours going from brunch with one friend to coffee with another, to visiting another friend's shop, just going with the flow. In the third trimester, I started to get more swelling in my legs, and it became harder to walk. I was easily wiped out after just one hour on my feet, and I had to slow down and spend more time at home resting. I felt frustrated and lame, like I was letting down my friends, and I honestly didn't know how I would occupy myself alone at home. I gave myself a couple of days to mope around the house and sulk until I felt like I was ready to let it go. To lift my spirits, I had to find something to keep me busy and help me feel social while I was stuck on the couch. I decided to focus on making a new Pinterest page for baby clothes, baby food, even articles on sleeping and breastfeeding, and invited all my friends to weigh in on my Pinterest page."

Without realizing it, this patient did a great job of using IPT's principles to manage her disappointment of having to slow down her socializing. Here are the steps she used that you can try when you're feeling stressed around an adjustment:

1. **Name what's upsetting you.** ("I had to slow down and spend more time at home resting.")

2. **Articulate the identity change.** How does this change specifically conflict with your familiar roles, routines, and relationships? ("I'm happiest when I'm out and about.")

3. **Acknowledge your distress and take the time you need to accept your feelings.** ("I felt frustrated and lame, like I was

letting down my friends, and I honestly didn't know how I would occupy myself alone at home—I gave myself a couple of days to mope around the house and sulk until I felt like I was ready to let it go.")

4. **Come up with a plan for how to adapt to your new circumstances.** ("I decided to focus on making a new Pinterest page . . . and invited all my friends to weigh in.")

It took this patient several weekends trying to stick to her old routine, and then crashing, before she could accept that her pace wasn't realistic anymore. For this patient, letting go of her busy Saturdays required mourning her independence before she could think of some practical steps to feel better in her new circumstances.

As helpful as IPT is for preventing depression, it cannot protect you from the grief you'll feel when saying goodbye to experiences that you'll never be able to exactly re-create. But that sadness, while unpleasant, isn't necessarily harmful. For most of us, it's the bottling up and denying of our feelings that is actually a greater trigger for depression than experiencing the gloom. Rather than pretending nothing has changed and forcing yourself to "power through it," IPT teaches you to acknowledge your disappointment and frustration in order to loosen up these emotions, which may help you to feel freer as you're trying out your new plan.

In order to figure out how you specifically can adapt to your new body and experiences, you'll have to open your eyes and take a hard look at your new circumstances. Yes, it's demanding to face all the changes demanded by your pregnancy and, soon, postpartum body and life, but if you don't look squarely at your new inner and outer world, you won't be able to figure out how to hold on to yourself along the way.

The Psychology of Your Third-Trimester Body

By now, you have already felt your baby's movement and even seen the skin on your belly pushed by a tiny hand or foot. For many, the strangeness and miracle of it are a delight. The physical experience may confirm that this must really be happening, which may deepen your emotional attachment. Some women wish they could share this bonding pleasure with their partner if he can't yet see and feel the baby from the outside. Some women feel exposed when they feel movements in public, as if others can see what's going on inside. **Others find it surreal; the fact that there's a tiny baby swimming around inside their body reminds them of a parasite, or the body invaders from** *Alien.*

Many women feel reassured by these sensations: Everything must still be okay in there if the baby is moving. While it isn't necessarily medically accurate, it's fine to make this assumption if it feels calming. But the flip side is that when the movements come and go, waiting for the next one may make you worry something is wrong.

One of our patients told us, "Early in my third trimester, I was walking down the stairs at the train station on my morning commute, and I realized I could no longer see my toes over my belly. I grabbed on to the rail in a panic—how could I safely go down stairs if I didn't know where my feet were?—and I walked so slowly the rest of the way down that I was holding up everyone behind me. I felt self-conscious and also a little pissed off that people were rushing me even though I was obviously hugely pregnant."

In the third trimester, your body may start to feel foreign to you. This goes beyond the way your shape changed in the second trimester. Even the most basic experiences, like how you walk down stairs, go to the bathroom, or tie your shoes, are transformed by your third-trimester body. Your body requires you to rethink your basic routines and pace, whether you're in an exercise class, at work, driving, or pushing a supermarket cart with a huge belly that's in the way. It can be difficult to accept that you can't continue at your usual speed, and you may be frustrated by your limitations.

While physical impediments are one problem, your body determines not just how you move but how you engage with the world. When your third-trimester body interrupts your social life with your friends or partner, we recommend that you do your best to explain how you're feeling, physically and emotionally, to the people in your life who are closest to you. This is both so they can understand the reasons you can't behave as you did, and so they can support you.

In one of our favorite scenes from *Sex and the City* (a show that worked to dispel sugarcoated myths about dating and marriage, in addition to pregnancy), Miranda is pregnant and audibly farts while at brunch with Carrie, Samantha, and Charlotte. "I'm pregnant; I can't control it," she says. Samantha responds, "Honey, you better learn, because that is unappetizing." Miranda keeps going: "I know. I am so swollen and gassy, I'm like a floatation device."

Miranda uses a combination of perfect comedic timing (it's a TV show, after all!) and unapologetic honesty to explain to her friends that in pregnancy, her body will do things that she can't always control. She's a bit annoyed and embarrassed, but because these are her best friends, she also feels safe enough to talk about a body experience that, at any other brunch, would be TMI. And she recognizes that the bar for TMI in pregnancy is just different. By informing them in a straightforward way, she's able to break down the barriers that most of us feel when talking about our bodies, even with the women we most trust.

Many women tell us they feel guilty when they "complain" about their pregnant bodies, because they also feel fortunate to be pregnant. But if you stop and think about it, complaining doesn't cancel out gratitude. The problem with a rule like "no complaining" is that it prevents you from releasing your negative thoughts and feelings—and talking about negative thoughts and feelings is often the fastest track to helping them go away. And if you don't talk about what's bothering you, you won't be able to benefit from the support of others.

You likely have friends who've struggled with similar pregnancy problems, and they can give you advice about how they and others have adjusted to the changes. Or you may have friends who've been through other dramatic body changes, perhaps resulting from a chronic illness or eating disorder, who can offer empathy and comfort. We believe that if women started sharing rather than keeping secrets about their bodies during pregnancy, it could normalize (and revolutionize) an experience that's been viewed as a source of embarrassment or shame.

One of our patients struggled with how embarrassing pregnancy symptoms distanced her from her friends. She told us, "Third-trimester hemorrhoids were absolutely the worst part of my pregnancy. Part of what was so hard about it is that I didn't tell anyone other than my doctor. I got into this huge fight with my best friend (who had never been pregnant) because I told her I couldn't come to her birthday dinner because I wasn't feeling well, and she freaked out. I felt guilty, frustrated, and was also really embarrassed."

Using IPT techniques, she realized that what felt like a shameful private medical issue was also putting stress on her pre-pregnancy identity as a generous and available friend. She realized that the best course of action was openness: "I decided to explain to her that I had hemorrhoids and that it was really painful to sit for long stretches without sitting on this special pillow—and the pillow was the kind of thing that I didn't want to carry around with me to a restaurant. Ultimately, telling her was a huge relief. Once she understood what I was going through, she understood that I wasn't just blowing her off. We both agreed that I should just stop by the dinner to say hi at the beginning but not stay for the whole party. It actually was kind of funny; she told me all about her sister's pregnancy hemorrhoids. I guess hemorrhoids are more common than I realized."

If you're embarrassed about sharing with a friend what feels like a shameful body issue, try to put yourself in her place. If a close friend told you she had hemorrhoids, would your reaction be "Ew, gross!"? Or would you instead express sympathy and ask what you could do to help your friend not be in pain? Often physical ailments that feel embarrassing are just like any other source of pain, and a good friend—or kind stranger—will respond with compassion, not disgust.

Accepting Your Unfamiliar Body

Another change that you'll undergo in the third trimester (if you haven't already) is the transformation in what you see when you look in the mirror. In the second trimester, you already started adjusting to the fact that you were gaining weight in order to grow a baby. As your pregnancy advances, that becomes more extreme. Rather than looking like a bigger version of yourself, you might start to feel like your body is unrecognizable.

You may be able to wear only a few items from your regular wardrobe. While some women love how maternity clothes make them feel, other women find themselves feeling disconnected from an aspect of self-expression that once reinforced their identity. **For most of us, our clothes reflect how we see ourselves (literally and psychologically) and how we want others to see us too.** Losing your usual wardrobe can be surprisingly painful.

One of our patients said, "When I started looking for maternity clothes and getting hand-me-downs from friends, I couldn't find anything that felt like 'me.' It felt awful at first. But then I rejected maternity clothing for a while and got creative, wearing my normal sweaters open and combining leggings and belts. Figuring out how to find the stretchy version of my normal look definitely helped my mood. Those matchy-matchy conservative 'mom-style' maternity clothes were just sad!"

This patient used an IPT approach to name the role change she was experiencing from having to change her wardrobe, reflect on how important her style was to her identity, and acknowledge the feelings she normally derived from her outfits. Rather than hold on to her old role (by forcing herself to squeeze into her old clothes) or deny how she was feeling (by wearing maternity clothes that were "not her"), she came up with a plan to preserve the identity she normally experienced from her style by adapting her new shape with some creative modifications. For her, figuring out a way to dress that suited her style helped her feel more in control of one significant way her identity was changing during pregnancy. Finding the right clothes was no profound insight, but for her, the psychological impact of continuing to feel good about her appearance was essential to preserving her self-esteem.

It may seem like these changes are superficial (by this we don't mean bad, just that changing your clothes is a surface-level intervention), but it might be helpful to think about what, from your usual appearance, you want to try to preserve during pregnancy. For this patient, it was her clothes; for another, it was continuing to make the time to style her hair in spite of feeling exhausted. For another, letting go of her time-consuming blow-dry was essential, and she felt great about getting a lower-maintenance shorter haircut. Every woman is different, and it's important to figure out what makes you feel confident and good.

Pregnancy in Public

Now that your bump is extremely obvious, your private self becomes, in some ways, a matter of public interest. With just one glance, any stranger will assume that you had sex and made a baby—very few times in life will you have so little privacy around an experience so profoundly private. Perhaps at another time in your life, you've received attention for revealing a visible tattoo, having a cast on a broken limb, or losing a significant amount of weight. But your external appearance likely hasn't revealed something as intimate as does your pregnant belly. And unlike a tattoo, by the time you're in the third trimester, your pregnant belly can't really be covered up.

Everyone feels different about the public aspect of her pregnant body. Some women feel beautiful and proud of their pregnant bodies and more confident about showing their shape than ever before. Others feel exposed and need more space and quiet to insulate themselves, even wearing headphones in public—playing music or not—to discourage strangers from engaging with them.

How much or how little attention you enjoy in public shows one aspect of how you feel about your personal boundaries. Just as you may not want to discuss religion, money, or politics with a casual acquaintance, you may feel that your pregnancy is an inappropriate topic to discuss in public, especially with someone you don't know well. Even a coworker's innocent "How are you feeling?" may make you uncomfortable, especially if you're *not* feeling well and are trying to keep your issues with acid reflux and ankle swelling out of the office lunchroom chat and off your mind while you're at work.

Some strangers' intrusions go beyond personal questions to physical touch. Almost every patient of ours has had at least one experience of a stranger touching her belly without asking permission. Some women experience this as a positive connection, and some laugh it off, but others feel violated. There's no wrong way to feel.

Why do so many people forget the normal rules of privacy when they're around pregnant women? A pessimistic reading of the situation would be that pregnancy erases a woman's individuality, and people start seeing her as a vessel for a baby. But there's a more positive framing: The pregnant body is a powerful symbol that evokes strong feelings from all of us—hope and power in bringing a new life into the world, or sentimental fondness reflecting back on the past. One of our patients shared how she experienced this: "On the days that people commented and I was in a good mood, I sort of felt like my pregnant body was somehow all of ours—new life, the future of the species—and that it made sense for everyone to be excited about it, like a universal positivity." Many will view you through the lens of "The Goddess Myth," which idealizes every pregnancy experience and every pregnant woman. They see you as an earth mother, calm and serene, generously tending to others—including attending to the emotional needs of strangers who stop you on the street.

Another patient described how she coped when approached during her third trimester: "I really didn't mind when random strangers talked to me. I am from a family of way too many opinions, so I am well accustomed to letting advice go in one ear and out the other. But touching my belly without asking was totally different. The first time it happened, I was so shocked I didn't say anything. So I made sure I had a line ready to go for the next time: 'No touching, please.' And yeah, there were plenty of next times."

Sometimes strangers' and acquaintances' comments on your pregnancy come in the form of comments on your appearance, which can also be challenging. Some women feel valued when strangers comment on their changing shape. One patient told us that when people on the street told her she was "looking great," it made her feel proud and appreciated. Another patient took the same compliment to mean that she didn't always look good before. One patient told us, "I hate when I hear women compliment each other by saying 'You're all belly,' because it's secret code that, aside from your belly, the rest of your body is still skinny. And that's not how my body handles pregnancy!" Another one of our patients told us, "My older son wasn't trying to be mean, but he genuinely said, 'I didn't know you could get pregnant in your butt,' because I had gotten so wide from behind. You can't control where you gain weight during pregnancy, and I just felt like a piece of meat when anyone commented on my body."

Your easily visible pregnancy may invite comments from strangers that aren't about your appearance but can leave you feeling equally judged. The barista may give you a dirty look when you ask for an extra shot of espresso. A waitress may shake her head in disapproval when you get fries instead of a side salad. Your aunt may comment on how tired you look, and recommend that you start your maternity leave before the baby arrives. Unsolicited comments may make you feel objectified, as if people are seeing you only as a "baby maker" rather than as an individual, and assuming that they know things about your life because of your appearance. They may suppose that just because you're pregnant, pregnancy is the only thing on your mind. But that assumption may be a reflection of what's happening in the other person's own mind. When you're pregnant, some people—old and young, men and women—will look at you and get sucked into a psychological portal where they can think about only their own feelings about the circle of life. No wonder their reactions to your body are so intense.

Unsolicited Advice

As one of our patients shared, "Every little old lady and middle-aged mom who stops me to talk acts like she has the best advice in the world on pregnancy and parenting. It's amazing how vividly women remember their pregnancies."

Why do some women (including other mothers) lose their advice filter when it comes pregnancy? Most are just trying to help. Some may be so moved by their own memories of pregnancy that they are simply not considering how their feedback might make you feel. Others may think they're inoculating you against bad luck or giving you a cold dose of reality to help you prepare. One of our patients told us, "My in-laws are not particularly positive, optimistic people, but it went into overdrive in my third trimester. Every time I saw them, it was 'It's going to be harder than you think!' and 'Enjoy sleep while you can!' I felt like they were trying to scare me or to justify how unhappy they'd been with their babies by convincing me I'd be unhappy with mine." Even when advice is intended to be helpful and constructive, the best intentions can't prevent you from feeling hurt.

Another patient told us that a friend came up to her at her baby shower to share the story of her emergency C-section. Yes, there was a happy ending where everything turned out well, but our patient did not particularly want to hear the frightening details, especially not in the middle of her party. Apparently, the friend wanted to share the story because she thought it might be helpful, since she herself tends to be calmed by thinking through worst-case scenarios in advance. Our patient had to explain to her friend that all this information was making her feel more stressed and out of control. She decided to protect her emotional boundaries by saying to her friend, "I know you're trying to be helpful, and that this was really hard for you, but I'd rather not talk about this right now—it stresses me out to imagine bad situations."

We encourage you to follow her lead and put up those boundaries with anyone who is approaching you with third-trimester TMI. When another woman shares her birth stories, she may think she's creating a bonding experience for the two of you, or offering knowledge she wishes she had. But it's okay for you not to experience the story in the same spirit.

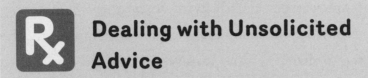

Dealing with Unsolicited Advice

If unsolicited comments and advice are making you feel powerless or irritable, consider this:

- **Remember, it's about THEM.** You can deflect from an intrusive person by asking them questions about their experiences. If a coworker tells you to stay off your feet because your ankles will get too swollen, you can say, "Oh, interesting, my feet have been feeling fine. Did your ankles bother you in your pregnancy?"

- **Browse but don't buy.** Try to think of unsolicited advice as window-shopping: You can observe it from afar, and maybe you'll come back and try it on, but there's no commitment.

- **Consider it preparation.** Unfortunately, some people feel just as free to comment on strangers' parenting as on their pregnancies. Learning how to distance yourself when you feel intruded upon is good practice for parenthood. You'll continue to deal with comments about everything from whether your child's coat is warm enough to his behavior in a restaurant.

- **Laugh it off.** You can use humor to mask more direct rebukes: "Mind the bump, please!" One of our patients would respond to strangers touching her belly by reaching her hand out and touching theirs. It amused her, and it showed them clearly how inappropriate their action was.

- **Speak up.** Practice a breezy "Okay, thanks!" and walking away. If you don't want to hear an upsetting story: "I'm sorry you went through that, but talking about this right now is stressing me out." If someone asks an intrusive question: "I'd rather not talk about that." And if people touch you without asking permission, you are well within your rights to tell them to stop.

Financial Planning and Your Partner

Couples enter parenthood with all sorts of financial arrangements. Some have been pooling their money in a joint bank account, some have separate bank accounts but share one credit card, some split everything fifty-fifty, and others have been entirely independent from each other. Of course, single moms and co-parents who aren't coupled have financial arrangements specific to them, too.

Now that your child will add a new wrinkle to your financial arrangements, it's likely that you'll have to reconsider not just your pre-parenthood budget but also your entire approach to finances. For some couples, these conversations occur in the third trimester, but some eager financial planners will have them far in advance.

We encourage you to start these discussions before the baby comes. Aside from the fact that clearheaded financial planning is nearly impossible to do in the presence of a crying newborn, your spending on baby care items begins well before the baby is born. The costs of clothes, diapers, health care, transportation, and child care (even if you're a stay-at-home mom, you'll need a babysitter on occasion) quickly add up.

Couples who are parents often find that their financial conflicts relate to time and child care. Now and for the next ten or more years, every time you want or need to do something without your child— work, a date with your partner or friends, an exercise class—you'll need to find someone to care for him, and most of the time that will involve paying someone.

You will have to decide what else is worth paying for. Will you pay someone to help you clean your home? Will you cook from scratch or spend money on takeout? You and your partner may have different ideas about when you should spend money for these services or spend the time doing it yourselves.

We recommend that you and your partner sit down now, if you haven't already, and decide how you're going to handle your baby-related expenses. Look carefully at your current credit card statements and bank accounts to assess how you've been spending your money pre-pregnancy. Then educate yourself (see **Resources**) about baby-related expenses and figure out what you can afford, where you have to make cuts, and who is going to pay for what.

Even if one of you feels like you're "bad at money" and would prefer the other partner to be in charge, we recommend that you consider making these financial decisions, which impact both of your lives, together. Aside from planning for new baby-related expenses, now is an important time to discuss any ongoing frustrations about your spending patterns. Do you resent your partner for paying for an expensive cable plan when he could cut costs by watching shows online? Does your gym membership (that you don't always use) bother your wife? Do you agree that staying in and cooking would save money, but you both hate cooking and resent the other for not taking the lead? Now is a good time to bring up these ongoing disagreements so that they're not exacerbated by the stress—financial and emotional—of a new baby. What feels practical and "fair" to each of you?

Going from Two Incomes to One

If you or your partner will be forgoing income to stay home with the baby, we recommend you discuss the following questions. They may be tough, but they're important.

- **How does the person who gives up a paycheck have access to funds?** For example, if you're a stay-at-home mom, you probably don't want to have to ask your partner for money to pay for personal items (the same is true for stay-at-home dads). Having to negotiate with your partner about how much you should spend on the moisturizer or jeans you've bought yourself for years can make you feel powerless and will no doubt put stress on your relationship. The nonearning person is still "working" for the family in terms of child care and will still need a voice in the small day-to-day purchases as well as the larger financial decisions. It may be helpful, even if you've always pooled all your finances, to give each partner a personal spending account separate from the family finances, which you can spend at your personal discretion.

- **How will you monitor your budget together?** If only one of you is the primary caregiver, does the less hands-on person get a say in baby-related spending? For example, if you're the one pushing the stroller most of the time, do you get to decide how much money to spend on a particular model, or does your partner also get input? If your partner is away at work most of the day and thinks that paying for a weekly babysitter while you're already home and not earning (so you can nap, exercise, or run errands) is a waste of money, how much say do you each get in this decision? By deciding this in advance, you can avoid future arguments about who's responsible for which parts of the family budget.

- **What about domestic work?** If one of you is going from working outside the home to being a stay-at-home parent, will that person also be expected to do all the cooking, cleaning, and laundry? How will your change in roles change your chores routine? Should the person working outside of the home take on more domestic responsibilities or child care on the weekend in order to give the primary caregiver a break?

Money may seem to be a practical aspect of your relationship, but it's also deeply psychological and rooted in other aspects of your individual identity. When you become parents, changes in the way you spend your money may impact your sense of routine, familiarity, and self. Because people vary in their psychological responses to spending, you and your partner are likely to have different emotions around this adjustment.

Your overall attitude about spending in your new family will probably connect back to feelings about how your childhood family handled finances when you were growing up. If your parents were careful about their budget and taught you well, you may be frustrated by your partner's money struggles. But if budgeting feels emotional, look at how you may be reacting to—or reacting against—your financial upbringing. Were your parents so thrifty that you never had an allowance for recreation, so now you want to enjoy your income instead of saving? Did growing up poor leave you with constant anxiety about your checking account, even after you secured a well-paying job? Did your parents constantly fight about money, leaving you afraid of talking about a budget with your partner at all?

If you and your partner end up fighting about money, ask yourself if you're working too hard to protect yourself from—or defend—the financial model you grew up with. You may end up too stubborn and unable to compromise if you're scared about repeating patterns or intent on resolving patterns you observed in childhood.

If you're feeling extra-sensitive, try to find a way to explain your fears to your partner so she can understand that it's anxiety, not anger or manipulation, behind your strong feelings about spending. Even if you two don't agree, you may be able to find some way to negotiate or at least learn more about each other's family histories so that you can empathize with your partner's financial pet peeves. It may be helpful to read the various recommendations of personal finance experts for an outside opinion or new ideas on how family finances can work. It's worth having these discussions now (hopefully ending with productive compromise) rather than once the baby is here and there's less money and more sleep deprivation.

Sometimes, in spite of the most responsible planning, financial stress is inevitable. For example, if you find yourself having difficulty with breastfeeding, you may want to hire a lactation consultant who wasn't in your original budget, or the cost of formula may hike up your grocery bill.

Other unpredictable financial events may be related to your

source of income. Because the childbearing years overlap with the time when most couples are building their careers, it's common to have unexpected work and income changes when you're a new parent, and we recommend talking through these potential challenges now.

One of our patients faced this early in her second pregnancy: "When I was pregnant with my second baby, our daughter was two years old. My husband and I both had new jobs. We thought the biggest headache would be my lack of maternity leave (being a new hire), but then, on the day of my fourteen-week doctor's appointment, my husband was fired. I still get this ache in my stomach to think about it. We decided to put off telling anyone he was fired, to avoid the social pressure on him. I was trying so hard to be supportive, but I was really stressed."

She ultimately decided to tell her family about her husband's unemployment, and her mother was able to come to stay with them to help take care of their older daughter after the baby was born. Her husband also decided that keeping the secret from his family wasn't worth it. Because their foundation of mutual support and communication (first just within their relationship, and later, involving their extended families) was strong, this couple was able to ride it out and recover from these financially—and emotionally—demanding circumstances.

If your own relationship with your parents is fraught, it may feel infantilizing to ask them for a loan, or you may be wary of opening yourself up to their criticism or invasive questions ("Why don't you have a job with better maternity leave?" or "Why can't your partner pay for this—is she struggling at work?"). You and your partner will need to decide together what sacrifices you'll make for financial stability. Of course, not all couples have families to fall back on financially in case of emergency. Some new parents are also financially supporting their own aging parents. The U.S. lags behind the rest of the developed world in maternal financial supports, but see our **Resources** for government-sponsored initiatives for pregnant women and families.

Friends and Family: Planning for Help in the Early Postpartum

The third trimester is a good time to start thinking about family assistance in child care, either temporary or ongoing. In many cultures, a woman's female relatives stay with her for days or weeks after childbirth while she recovers. For many families in the U.S., this isn't a given, but it can still be a good option for many mothers. If you have a good relationship with your mother, mother-in-law, or other women in your family, and if they are available and haven't already volunteered, you may want to ask them to stay with you or visit after the baby is born. (Of course, this can apply to any helpful, trusting relatives or very close friends, including uncles and fathers.) Don't feel that you need to wait for them to offer, and don't take their lack of volunteering as reluctance. In our experience, some grandparents prefer to wait to be asked (to both feel wanted and, in the best of circumstances, respect your boundaries). And some won't anticipate that you'll need hands-on help but can rally if you directly ask.

It's possible they haven't offered because they're not interested or able, and they'll either say no or reluctantly agree (and perhaps passive-aggressively sabotage the offer by, for example, "getting sick" on their babysitting day). There's no way to predict if or how they'll be supportive, but it certainly helps for you to be as specific as possible when you ask for what you need, and to make sure your request or invitation leaves room for them to decline or to choose a different, less demanding way to be supportive. Waiting for your family to read your mind (so you don't feel guilty about being too pushy) will just lead to miscommunication and disappointment.

Before the baby arrives, some extended families may make an unsolicited offer to new parents for help in terms of money or other forms of hands-on assistance (babysitting, cooking meals, etc.). This can be supportive practically but complicated psychologically if it comes with implicit obligations or emotional strings attached. If your mother is babysitting every Wednesday, does she expect a weekly briefing on all of your parenting decisions? Or do you have a feeling she won't respect your decisions and will go rogue? If your eccentric aunt offers to come stay with you for a week, will her presence put too much of a strain on your relationship, or do you anticipate needing to play hostess? If the emotional cost of accepting these offers of financial help or labor is too high, and you can survive without it, don't be afraid to say no. If you accept, make sure you are very clear with your family about your understanding of the emotional implications that may accompany the gift or loan.

You and your partner may have different points of view in terms of help from family members. One of our patients wanted her mother to stay with her and the baby after she came home from the hospital. She knew her mother would be happy to take on some of the chores, like laundry and cooking, while offering support and advice. Her husband felt hurt when she suggested this plan, because he thought this would be bonding time for them with the baby. While our patient liked the spirit behind his suggestion, she also knew that her husband wasn't the best cook, and she worried that she would end up feeling exhausted by the housekeeping that he might not keep up with. She explained to him that while her mother might interrupt some of their new-family bonding time, her mother's help could also open up time for them to enjoy the baby by helping out with the domestic work that her husband wasn't used to being in charge of. Her husband was reluctant, but our patient promised that she would cut the visit short if her mother's presence was causing more harm than good, and she made sure that her mother was up for a flexible end date, too. They agreed that this was a better plan than refusing her support.

If you or your partner decide that you don't want family around, or your family isn't available, consider saving up and hiring some help, to give you a break to get to a doctor's appointment, run errands, or catch up on sleep.

If hired help is not affordable, consider asking other mothers in your neighborhood what they do when they're having a sick day or need any assistance with their babies. In some communities, there are parents who trade off in supporting each other, parents who come together to hire a shared child care professional (aka "nanny share") and other flexible or creative options. Caring for a baby is exhausting, and you will need an occasional break, even if it's just for an hour or two. The benefits of a break are not only practical but also psychological, as being responsible for a vulnerable infant 24/7 is too heavy a load for anyone to carry without burning out.

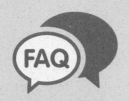 The following are some common questions we hear from women in the third trimester:

Should I have a baby shower?

Baby showers are not a ritual in every religion and culture. If a shower is not part of your cultural tradition, you should ask people to respect that and save celebrations and gifts for after the baby's arrival, or to adapt however you prefer.

Though a cynical economist may suggest that baby showers and registries are a cultural manipulation to get us to "buy more stuff," in the best of worlds, they are supportive in more ways than one. Baby showers are a ritual for your community to come together and show support for you during this happy and challenging transition. Transitions between identities and phases in life fall into the category of what anthropologists call "liminality." It's a state of in-between, ambiguity, and passing through. Because liminal times are emotionally exhausting, cultures develop rituals or rites of passage to support people during these phases. Baby showers are one of these rituals.

Your baby shower can be your chance to let your community support you. On a practical level, shower registries can take financial pressure off expectant parents by providing some of the supplies a new baby requires. And the showers themselves can be a fun excuse to party before the work of taking care of a newborn arrives. By surrounding you with a comforting community of women—or people of all genders—whom you can call on for advice and support, a shower reminds you that you are not alone.

As with most family gatherings, baby showers can be stressful. If your sister-in-law considers the occasion an opportunity to show off her new home, or your mother decides to pick a fight with your aunt about whether to serve alcohol, you can end up surrounded by a group of people who are more focused on their own worries and needs than yours, leaving you feeling disappointed in your support system. There's no way to gather three to a hundred people (especially your relatives) in a room without encountering some who make you happy and others who push your buttons.

Even if you don't really want a shower, you might want to say yes to family or friends who are eager to host one. Maybe you'll agree to let your mother's best friend throw you a shower simply because your mother wants her to. Sometimes in life we make decisions to honor the feelings of the people we love. If that's your reason for agreeing to a shower, just remind yourself that you're doing it for them, not you, in any moment when you may be feeling annoyed by the experience. And you might end up pleasantly surprised: Even if you don't love a party, you might enjoy your shower when you see how happy it makes your mother (or sister or best friend).

In the end, a baby shower is optional. Sometimes not wanting a shower is simply a case of the introvert/extrovert divide. If you feel self-conscious being the center of attention, or drained by large gatherings of people, you might find the whole thing an exhausting burden and prefer to go out with your two best friends and mom for an intimate brunch. One first-time mother whose extended fam-ily lived on the other side of the country explained how she made compromises in planning her shower: "I had a small shower that was mostly just my friends. I felt like it would make things too much of a big deal to ask my family to get on a plane again, especially just to watch me eat and open gifts."

It can help you to think about the type of party that would make you the happiest. Remember, if you agree to have a shower, you don't have to be a passive participant. Speak up about what you want and don't want. You can limit the guest list to only those you really want there. You can say no games, or no gifts outside of the registry, please, or no gifts at all. One of our patients made these modifications: "We had a shower, but not a traditional one. Instead of a women-only brunch or tea, we decided to plan a casual coed Saturday-night party in our living room for our best friends—no family—with music and alcohol. We said no gifts because it just felt wrong to ask friends who are on tight budgets to buy things for us. We just wanted to have a party, knowing that it would be much harder to see people after the baby was born, and building a bridge between our pre-baby social life and our future as parents."

If you're not comfortable asking people to buy you gifts but are unable to afford your baby gear without assistance, you can ask moms in the group to bring any hand-me-downs they want to loan or pass on. Not only does this save everyone from the expense, but you'll get to see what your friends really used and liked best with their babies. One of our patients explained, "Most of my friends and cousins are already moms with older kids, so they brought me stuff they had used and loved. It gave me confidence knowing that these were blankets, gear, and onesies cherished by others. Using their hand-me-downs made me feel welcomed into the community."

Many women tell us that they find registering to be overwhelming because there are so many choices for different variations of baby products on the market. Others enjoy the research, which makes them feel informed and prepared. You can do research online or ask mothers you know and trust. Remember that if you don't register, some friends and family may still buy you gifts—just gifts of their own choosing. Do your best to make your desires and expectations clear.

Is the "nesting urge" a real thing?

One way you may begin to connect with your baby is by building a protective environment. You may start transforming your home—decorating a nursery, or simply cleaning out closets or drawers to make space. You may also begin to piece together a community of people who make you feel safe and supported, and distance yourself from people you don't trust. In a sense, this helps you build a social "nest" where you and your new family can feel safer, settled, and supported.

Some pregnant women feel the urge to reorganize or decorate their home (in general, not only the baby's room) in a way that is not just practical but feels propelled by strong emotion. Sometimes nesting urges are quirky or obsessional (this may be related to the same triggers that cause women with a history of obsessive-compulsive disorder to have a flare in their symptoms during pregnancy). If you head to the kitchen for midnight ice cream and end up on your hands and knees reorganizing the freezer drawers until they look "just right," you may have been struck by the nesting urge. Studies have shown that nesting often takes hold in bursts of energy that break through even the exhaustion of the third trimester.

There are hormonal components to the nesting urge (in animals, scientists think that nesting behavior involves prolactin, a hormone also used in producing milk, as well as estrogen and progesterone). Nesting is also psychological. It's a time-honored coping mechanism, a way to assuage anxiety by controlling what you can (your immediate environment) in the face of an unpredictable future. Fathers and nonpregnant partners may also feel the urge to prepare for the baby's arrival. However, the passionate nesting inspired by pregnancy may put you at odds with your partner. Some of our patients have told us about feeling a powerful drive to organize their entire home, but their partner was more laid-back, and these differences were frustrating. Do your best to communicate clearly about what you're feeling, and to ask for what you need instead of waiting for your partner to be magically inspired. As with any hormonally inspired feelings, remember that the urgency you feel has physiological and emotional origins—it's not only about the state of your home.

Depending on the other demands on your time, or if your baby arrives early, you may not get everything arranged or ordered to your satisfaction. If you find yourself in that situation and feel panicked, try to remind yourself that much of this anxiety is driven by feeling out of control because of the emotional shifts of matrescence. Organizing your home may be soothing but is only a superficial way to feel more in command of a time that will be psychologically messy no matter how perfect your sock drawers look.

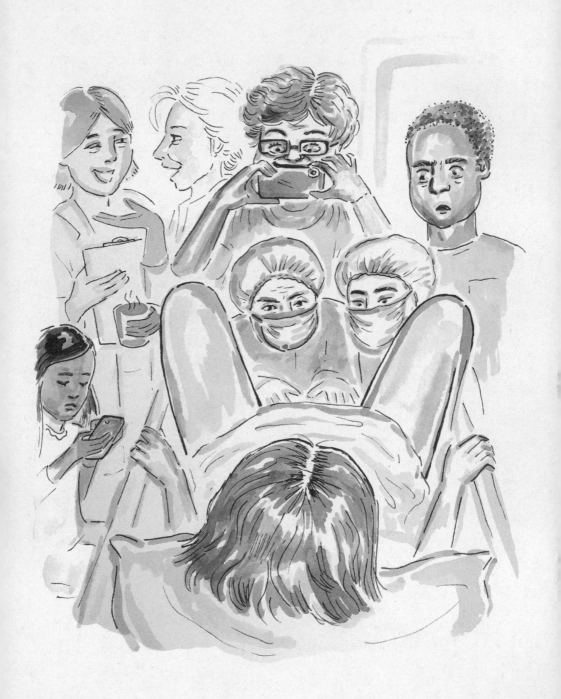

Labor and Delivery

Preparing for the Emotional Ride of Childbirth

Childbirth is simultaneously one of life's most natural and super-natural experiences. Rationally, we know that our bodies are built to give birth. But the logistics of growing a human in your body, then pushing it out your vagina and into your arms, sound more like the stuff of science fiction—or horror—than real life. You may intellectually understand that you are about to deliver a baby, but—as with mortality—you may find it difficult to fathom emotionally.

Even when you try to wrap your head around what's about to happen, giving birth may be impossible to imagine if you've never experienced it. You may have expectations for how it will go, but these are desires and wishes as much as they are plans. To sort out the feelings that may swirl between fantasy and reality, it helps to reflect on how you've imagined childbirth over time and how the birth narratives you've heard may be shaping your expectations. Maybe you have a cousin who described natural birth as the best thing that ever happened to her, or a sister who loves to evangelize about epidurals, or you know someone who had a harrowing medical complication.

Culture also informs our ideas about childbirth. Maybe you've held on to the charmingly chaotic humor of Katherine Heigl in *Knocked Up* and expect that childbirth will be a romantic bonding experience with both your new baby and your partner. Or maybe you were traumatized by a tragic news story. Maybe the award-winning documentary *The Business of Being Born* left you feeling more educated but also terrified of being bullied by the medical system.

Even with today's medical options, you can't control every detail around how, when, where, and with whom your labor and delivery will unfold. So, given how much will remain unknown, how do you prepare yourself—emotionally—for childbirth?

There's no singular "right" way to feel about childbirth. As in the moment you found out you were pregnant, or any of the "big reveals" of pregnancy, panic is just as common as excitement. For many women, the giddy eagerness is electric: *After years of waiting for and months of feeling my baby from the inside, I'm finally going to meet her!* For others, there's eager anticipation for the end of physical discomfort: *Get this thing out of me!* Mixed in with this myriad of feelings is usually some nervousness, which, for some women, blends into fear or even dread. We can reassure you that trepidation about childbirth has no correlation with an increased risk of problems during birth. **It's perfectly natural to worry about one of the biggest events of your life, especially because so much of it is out of your control.**

Some women deal with the massive unknowns of childbirth by accepting that there's no foolproof way to prepare. These people are emotionally comforted by a "less is more" approach: They may use healthy (or, at times, unhealthy) forms of a defense that we call "denial" to avoid worrying about hypothetical problems until there is a concrete problem that they can fix. "Denial" isn't literal here— less-is-more people don't believe that childbirth won't happen if they don't think about it, but they do find it easier and less stressful to just not think about it. If thinking through potential outcomes just makes you feel worse, then you may want to skip the next section of this chapter, where we'll be describing and normalizing some of the most common fears of childbirth.

Other women feel soothed by thinking through all possible scenarios, even the most catastrophic. People with this type of psychology may use a different type of healthy (and, at times, unhealthy) defense: intellectualization. If you're in this group, you like to look your fears in the face and intellectually anticipate the unknown future, as scary as those hypotheticals may be. Parsing out your worries can feel like turning on a light when you've been in a dark room and are feeling spooked. If planning for the worst helps you feel more prepared, then this next section may provide a feeling of comfort and strategy.

It's Normal to Feel Nervous: The Most Common Anticipatory Fears of Childbirth

Most women, whether they admit it or not, experience fear mixed in with all the eager expectations of childbirth. Who wouldn't be anxious about an extreme physical task that they've never gone through? Isn't everyone at least a little intimidated before they run a marathon? It's human to ask yourself: What if I don't have what it takes?

Add to the physical intimidation that the stakes are much higher than finishing a race—in fact, they are literally life-and-death. We encourage you to remember that, on some level, everyone feels that way. If you're freaked out, we recommend you find your own calming mantras, or feel free to borrow ours: **1) Nervous is normal, and 2) Fear is just a feeling.**

We've found that it helps our patients when we validate how common most fears are and then remind them that anxiety about childbirth does not foreshadow any actual problems with childbirth. In other words, imagining a worst-case scenario does not have any correlation with a bad thing happening to you down the road, it just means that you have a vivid (and, likely, exhausting) imagination.

Some people experience worry in the form of physical tension, pain, or a pounding heart. Fear can make it hard for you to sleep, eat, or focus at work. Thoughts of danger can trigger your body's fight-or-flight response, pumping adrenaline through your veins and raising your heart rate and blood pressure. If you're feeling this way, we recommend you first try to calm your nervous system before indulging your thoughts. Breathing, meditation, yoga, massage, or a pleasant, distracting activity like time with friends or zoning out with TV or a book can help to remind your body and brain that even though you're imagining a terrifying situation, you're not currently in any danger.

Once you've found a way to chill out enough to think straight, it may help to start describing your fears to someone you trust or in your journal. Sometimes naming worries helps to tame them. That specificity can help you feel more in control, and to see how your fears about labor relate to other scary experiences you've made it through. In our experience, pre-labor fears tend to fall into the following categories:

Fear of Pain

You've probably received a lot of mixed messages about what giving birth actually feels like: "It's hell. Bad enough that I'd never consider getting pregnant again" versus "It's glorious and majestic—I've never felt more in touch with my strength and power" versus "You just have to get through it and won't remember much of it anyway" versus "Just take the drugs and let the doctors do the rest." If you, like many people, are scared of the feeling of extreme pain, remember that modern medicine has a lot of ways to help you—and that there's nothing wrong with using medication and technology to help your labor be less painful. One patient told us, "I felt 75 percent of my fear of childbirth fade away once I decided to plan on an epidural. I knew things could go wrong, and there were still so many unknowns, but it was a huge relief to know that the physical pain would be managed by my doctor." **Numbing the pain of childbirth does not make you any less of a woman; it's just a decision about creating the best birth experience for you.**

If you'd prefer not to use medication, there are many rituals that have helped women survive childbirth since (literally) the beginning of humankind. Most of these techniques involve breath, visualization, and other forms of mind and body work—a birthing class or work with a doula can be a great way to learn about these methods (see **Resources**).

One of our patients said, "No matter how terrified you are about the pain, try to remember that, unlike other types of pain in pregnancy (hemorrhoids, back pain), the pain of childbirth—at least physically—is intense but, in a way, temporary. The healing takes time, but for me, the pain didn't stick around for too long. And, unlike most pain in life, it doesn't mean anything is wrong. It means something powerful is happening. I used a mantra—'pain with a purpose'—because I knew it would lead me to my baby."

Fear of Losing Control

Childbirth is an ancient, primal part of life—which adds intensity to the experience greater than any you may have experienced before. **If you're used to finding comfort in control and planning, childbirth is going to take you out of your element.** Your body and the baby's will be doing things you can neither predict nor regulate. Birth plans (which we'll discuss later in this chapter) are useful tools, but they're not a promise, and they certainly won't guarantee your spot in the driver's seat.

One of our patients, who is a doula herself, shared her dream of a home birth and a fear of "failing at my innate abilities as a woman to give birth naturally." To her, a natural birth was central to her values and identity, and she feared that medical intervention would feel like losing herself and everything she believed in. It helped her to reflect on the pressure that she was putting on herself. Even this childbirth professional needed reminders that the body sometimes has a mind of its own, which helped her keep perspective.

For some women, fear of losing control during childbirth may be particularly profound if it is tied to past experiences of physical, sexual, or emotional trauma. Spreading your legs for a roomful of strangers who may not always explain what they are doing or ask you for permission can trigger memories for some women of the most violent encounters of their lives. If you find yourself thinking about past traumatic experiences, even if they are seemingly unrelated to your genitals and sexual history, we recommend talking about these worries with your birth provider as a part of your pre-birth process. There may be choices you can make in your birth plan to help yourself feel safer: *Do you want to plan for a midwife or ob-gyn practice that is all female? Do you want to require everyone who comes into your room to ask permission before touching you? Do you want to find a doula who is trained in working with women who have a history of trauma?* Later in this chapter, we'll continue the conversation on trauma as it relates to labor and delivery. While your plan can never be set in stone, it's a valuable opportunity to discuss your needs and desires with your practitioner.

Fear of Embarrassment

For some women, the fear of the pain of childbirth is nothing compared to the fear of the profound exposure—naked in stirrups, sweaty and screaming, gushing with bodily fluids and even bowel movements. For most women, there are only brief moments like this during the entire labor and delivery journey, but they still happen. Whether you're worried about feeling embarrassed because someone hears you cursing at your partner or because they see your poop or pubic hair, remember that the delivery room is exempt from the usual rules of social politeness. **When it comes to doctors, midwives, and other professionals, there's nothing they haven't seen before.** And if you're worried about what your partner will see, read on—we'll give you some more advice about how to discuss these concerns in advance of your labor to help you both feel more reassured.

In the end, for most women, childbirth has a wonderful way of making you forget your embarrassment in the moment. One typically buttoned-up patient said, "By the time I was actually in the stirrups, I didn't care at all about being naked. And I'm someone who wouldn't even change my gym clothes in front of my mother. But the last thing on my mind was my modesty—I just wanted my baby." And yes, because bowel movements while pushing are sometimes what women worry about most, we've heard countless patients say the same thing. Trust us, in the moment, neither you nor anyone in the room cares. You're busy pushing out a baby, and that's what everyone is thinking about.

Fear of Medical Intervention

Whether you're planning a home birth, scheduling a C-section, or aiming for anything in between, you may be afraid of interventions and complications that can happen during childbirth. Some women are just anxious about hospitals and hate the idea of spending time in them. Other women find themselves dwelling on potential complications: What if something goes wrong?

We recommend you talk to your practitioner about these fears. You can learn how rare emergencies are and talk about how your practitioner handles them. If you're planning a home birth, you can talk to your midwife about what happens if you face complications. She can educate you on the chances of needing to go to the hospital—and the helpfulness of doing so if the need arises.

If you're dreading spending time in the hospital, remind yourself that while you may go into your hospital delivery focused on the birthing experience, you'll leave with entirely different concerns about the baby and your healing. And everyone at the hospital shares your main goal: a healthy birth and a healthy baby. Your birth probably won't go perfectly, but on the other side of the experience, you may not be so preoccupied with the disappointments. Of course, you have the right to be angry and critical about anything related to your body and care, but we also think it's a beneficial exercise in gratitude to remind yourself that if you're going home with a healthy baby and no medical complications, this is a good outcome. As one patient of ours described: "I think people have this idea that hospitals are evil and push you into doing things you don't want to do—that's just not how it was for me. The hospital isn't like a spa or a feel-good spiritual center, but it is designed to protect you and your baby to the fullest, and that made me feel super-safe. I liked the fact that medical professionals were in control and I could just focus on myself and trust that they were in charge."

Fear of Helplessness and of Asking for Help

Being a hospital patient makes most of us feel helpless—you're physically exposed, and big intimidating institutions are difficult to navigate even when you're at your best. **It's common to feel like just a number.**

But for as many negative stories about interactions with hospital staff during moments of needing support, we've heard just as many positive stories. One of our patients told us about the bond she developed with the labor and delivery nurse who helped walk her to the bathroom during childbirth and in the early hours after: "I felt so tired, embarrassed, helpless, scared, and shaky—but my nurse was so patient, walking me to the bathroom and waiting there with me, with support. It was a relief knowing she was there and hearing her reassurance that this was normal, since she'd seen thousands of women go through this."

Unfortunately, we do hear stories about disappointing, even devastating, hospital experiences that would make anyone feel alienated, neglected, sad, and angry. In some cases, financially pressed hospitals put pressure on their staff to err on the side of efficiency rather than nurturing, but that's never an excuse for bad bedside manner.

One of the most painful and frustrating aspects of being a patient in the hospital is when you aren't able to control your own daily schedule. As one woman explained, "Every morning, the whole medical team—the med students, nurses, everybody—just showed up in my room at six a.m. and turned the lights on without even asking if I was sleeping. I had just finished feeding my baby twenty minutes before, and I'd finally gotten to sleep. I felt like they didn't care at all what I needed, just what their schedule was." Hospitals have some rules that may be out of everyone's control, but you can always ask for a change in schedule, for information, for more time with your doctor or nurse, and for more physical and emotional support.

Fear of the Unknown

Finally, remember that all these fears are about a wild, entirely un-predictable ride. It's kind of like the feelings of fear you may have at the beginning of a new relationship or new job: Often, both the worst and best parts of the experience are the most unplanned. If you can reframe your anxiety as anticipation or remind yourself that worrying won't help you prepare, you may be able to let go of some of the more negative ruminations. At some point in the relatively near future—a week or a month down the line—you'll know how your birth went. There's nothing to do but make it to that point, and trust that you will be able to make it and process your experience later.

It may also help to remind yourself how lucky you are to be living in an era when medical technology, while imperfect and at times unaffordable or administered by doctors with disappointing bedside manner, is more advanced than ever. If your baby has a medical need, there hopefully will be a treatment that can help. If you have a physical issue like vaginal tearing, there will be special-ists you can go to for help in your recovery. And, of course, there are many effective treatments for any emotional or psychiatric issues that may arise.

Try not to fear things "going wrong" during your labor and delivery; try to trust that the team you have assembled is trained and prepared to help. In a system that won't always ask you what you want, your only job is to speak up about the help you need.

You don't have to have a perfect childbirth in order to come out of the experience—eventually—feeling healthy, healed, and whole.

Another gratitude exercise that will help balance your fears is to remind yourself how lucky you are to be healthy enough to give birth—not everyone is able to. Furthermore, you're simply lucky to be alive. The most basic human experiences (creating life, feeling love, saying goodbye to people and experiences) all involve some difficulty and angst, and come with both pain and privilege. Sometimes we can get so focused on what we don't have that we forget to look at what's right in front of us. You and your baby made it through childbirth, and that's worth celebrating and honoring.

The Logistics: Hospital Tours, Birth Classes, and Birth Plans

One of the most important choices you'll have to make is who will deliver your baby. If you trust that person's overall values, communication skills, and judgment, you'll more likely agree with her decision-making in real time. You might be more comfortable with a no-nonsense ob-gyn, while your best friend might prefer a holistically educated midwife. Your choice of where to give birth—hospital, birthing center, or at home—is also significant, because the details of your birth are determined by the options at the setting you choose. You can't deliver by water birth in many hospitals, and it's unlikely that you'll be able to get an epidural if you deliver at home.

If you're delivering outside your home, you may be offered a tour of the center or hospital where you plan to give birth. Think of this as an opportunity to get yourself oriented to the practical details in advance: which entrance you should use, where your partner should park the car, and where to give your insurance information. Educating yourself about these little things can help you feel more in control and less stressed if your water breaks at three-thirty a.m. and there's no one in the lobby. Even if you're having a scheduled induction or C-section, it's one less thing you have to think about on an already stressful day.

Some women and their partners sign up for a childbirth education class in the third trimester. If you're unpartnered, you can go with the person you've asked to be your labor and delivery partner (more on that later) or by yourself. You may find the class both interesting and helpful, and enjoy the shared experience with your partner and others at the same life stage. On the other hand, you may be put off by the idea of talking about such an intimate experience in a room with strangers. If you are squeamish but your partner isn't, he can still get a lot out of the class without you, or vice versa. Or you can get the same information through books, documentaries, and online classes (see **Resources**).

If you're a "less is more" kind of person, the information overload in one of these classes might make you feel more anxious— the opposite of what you need. While you might feel that it's irresponsible not to "prepare" for your delivery, we'd like to remind you that women have been giving birth for millions of years without any curricula. **We encourage you not to think of labor as an exam you have to study for but as an experience in which your body and practitioner will lead the way.**

One of the most useful things to come out of birthing classes, either in person or online, can be a birth plan. Like taking a birthing class, writing a birth plan is not mandatory, but it may help you feel like you have a little more agency in this chaotic experience. And it may leave you with fewer decisions to make in the midst of labor.

In fact, it may be helpful to call this list your "birth preferences," which leaves you some more room to think about how you might want to handle different scenarios. You can't control the unknown, but you can prepare yourself for the choices you'll have—and get some of the decision-making done ahead of time. Therefore, the first step in writing your birth plan isn't deciding what you want but educating yourself and reflecting on your options with your partner. You may want to begin by asking your provider about the range of possibilities at the facility where you're delivering.

We encourage you to practice using language with yourself that is both assertive and flexible when thinking about your birth plan—this helps you advocate for yourself while leaving room for the unknown and uncontrollable aspects of birth. If you go into childbirth with all-or-nothing, judgmental rules, you're only setting yourself up to be disappointed when those strict rules have to be bent or broken.

How to Write a Wise Birth Plan

Here are a few examples of how to move from black-or-white thinking to a more flexible point of view when considering what kind of birth you want:

1. **Black-or-white:** "A natural birth is best."

   Flexible: "I want an unmedicated birth. I'll prepare with breathing classes, my doula will help me, and I'll explain to my doctor that I don't want an epidural. But if I ultimately ask my doctor for medication, that's okay—it may turn out that I needed it."

2. **Black-or-white:** "C-sections happen because the medical system is corrupt."

   Flexible: "I do not want to have to have a C-section for anyone's scheduling purposes or hospital discharge plans. However, if I need a C-section to protect my health or my baby's, of course I'll have one, and I won't blame myself."

3. **Black-or-white:** "This is my body and my child, and no one knows better than I do about what I need."

   Flexible: "This is my body and my child, and no one knows better than I do about what I *want*. But part of why I'm involving a health care/birthing professional is to advise about what I and my baby may *need*. They already know what I want, and I trust they will do their best."

Try to think of a birth plan as more a list of priorities or guidelines than a guaranteed blueprint of how your delivery will go. As one patient advised: "Write a birth plan, even if the first thing you do is throw it out when you get to the hospital. It helps you emotionally prepare for the crazy experience of childbirth. It can help focus your intention, too—an act that I think is worthwhile no matter how you end up delivering." Birth plans are a helpful framework for discussions with your practitioner as well. But once you've done all that work to clarify what you want, you will ultimately have to accept that birth plans, like due dates, are not binding, and getting too attached to either one can result in disappointment.

You can also put a plan B or a plan C in your birth plan. For example, if you're planning to use breathing techniques instead of pain medication to get through the contractions, great. But if breathing isn't enough, you can include massage and heat/cold packs as plan B and leave medication as an option for plan C. You can also specify which pain medications you'd prefer.

You may want to forgo a birth plan altogether; you can have a general conversation with your practitioner and otherwise just show up. Another option is to make some big-picture decisions but avoid worrying about the details, like this patient, who explained: "I told my doctor not to give me a C-section or contraction medications just to speed things up—I only wanted those if medically necessary. But otherwise, my birth plan was to just come out with a healthy baby."

However detailed you want your birth plan to be, you should discuss it with your provider, since she'll know more about your options and will have her own expertise to contribute. Once you've found out your options, you can sit down—by yourself, with your partner, or with a trusted friend—to think through what you want. While no birth plan is set in stone, you should think about what matters to you most in your birth experience: Do you prioritize minimizing pain, or do you want the full physical experience of a medication-free childbirth? Do you want your partner or doula to take decision-making pressure off you, or do you want to call the shots?

You should ask your practitioner what happens when the birth doesn't go according to plan. Sometimes on-the-fly decisions need to be made. One element of a birth plan is figuring out how those decisions happen. One patient told us, "I'd been in labor for thirty hours with little progress, and my epidural was only partly working. I just wanted things to be over, but I didn't know what the best thing was in that moment, and I was in no shape to decide if I wanted a C-section when my doctor asked me. I appreciate that they were empowering me, but I really wish someone had just told me, 'You need a C-section.' I kind of just wanted to ask her, 'What would you do? What would you do if this were your sister?'"

You can ask your practitioner ahead of time what they prefer to do for decisions that aren't life-or-death, and you can ask them to give you guidance, more or less. Another patient told us, "When my midwife said, 'I think you need an episiotomy,' I trusted her to make that decision. I knew she wouldn't suggest it unless it was really necessary."

By writing down your goals and talking to your care providers, you can confirm that they will do their best to help you have a birth that follows your priorities. If your practitioner is unable to make certain promises, ask her to clearly explain the rationale, and if that doesn't work for you, consider researching other professionals who may be better suited for you.

Your Partner and Birth

One of the decisions you have to make about your birth is who will be with you during birth. We recommend picking the person (or people) you trust most when you're at your most vulnerable, and who makes you feel the most comfortable so that you can focus on your own experience rather than being distracted by their needs.

For most women, that will be their spouse or partner. But how can you know in advance what your partner will be like in the delivery room if you've never been through anything like this together? That's one of the reasons we encourage both of you to learn about labor and delivery through classes you attend or videos you watch together during your pregnancy—in addition to being informative, they may provide clues about how your partner will react when the day arrives. You may be pleasantly surprised; even if she's usually squeamish at the sight of blood, you might see that she can be stoic when she needs to be.

As one of our patients told us: "I thought my husband would have a hard time being supportive emotionally. He's not used to being a caretaker. He's also easily grossed out, so I thought he would be making faces the whole time. I was surprised that he handled it much better than I would have expected. He really rallied and wasn't focused on himself at all—I had never seen him be that supportive, actually, but I think because we were really scared, we had to come together."

Ideally, your partner can also be your advocate, reminding your medical team about your wishes and concerns, both during labor and delivery and after the baby is born. He can be there with you not just physically but emotionally. He can let you know how much he loves you and what a great job you're doing. He can put aside—or at least appear to put aside—his own fears and focus on you. And he can understand that whatever you say during an intense contraction shouldn't be taken personally.

One patient advised trying to be as specific as possible with your partner about how you'd like him to be supportive. "I think you and your partner should come up with the ten commandments of what you will agree on to protect each other from everyone else's needs once the baby is born. Details. Nitty-gritty. Like, I wanted a free pass on anything I said during labor, even if it was really mean."

Think about how to set your partner up for success as your labor coach. Does your partner get cranky if she hasn't eaten in a couple of hours? Throw snacks for her in your go bag. Is she unable to function without a full night's sleep? Bring a pillow and an eyeshade for her to power-nap in case your labor lasts over twenty-four hours. It may make you feel resentful that you have to anticipate your partner's needs when you're the one on the hot seat, but try to remember that just because her job pales in comparison to yours, that doesn't mean she's invulnerable.

When it comes to making plans for the birthing room, there's always the chance that you and your partner will disagree on how things should happen. Of course, it's your body going through the labor—at the end of the day, you pretty much get to call the shots. But as you may have done in pregnancy, you should think about beginning to unite as teammates. One of our patients told us, "I wanted a home birth—I think of hospitals as a place for illness—but the idea of a home birth made my husband very anxious. We were able to find a birthing center that's affiliated with a hospital but is separate, and I found a midwife who was able to help me have the comfortable birth I wanted. It was a compromise that worked for both of us."

Including your partner in decision-making can help you feel less alone in the process. It can also be a way to invite him into the co-parenting process. Childbirth is one of the most drastic examples of moments in a relationship where one partner may feel less essential. Because there are so many biological setups for couples to feel this way, we encourage you to include your partner in those most basic separate experiences, because that will establish the structure of your parenting as a team with more equality. By indicating that your partner's values are important, you're also saying, "I couldn't do this without you, and this baby and the work of it are also yours."

Of course, there are obstacles to seamless teamwork. In labor and delivery, your partner may be observing the most intimate parts of your body in a way that is entirely unsexual, which can bring up complicated feelings and concerns for both of you. You may be concerned that he'll never desire you in a sexual way again, even if he is visibly in awe of what you're doing. These anticipatory fears are common, but in the heat of the moment, they're usually not what either of you will be focusing on.

Is your partner concerned that he'll never be able to look at you the same way again after he sees the baby's head emerge from your vagina? A patient told us that she worried when she saw the look on her wife's face as they watched a birthing video. She sat down with her wife in the third trimester and said, "Babe, I know you want to be supportive, but I don't want to see you grossed out when I'm trying to focus on delivering the baby. If I'm worrying about never being able to feel sexy again, that's just not helpful. You don't have to be a hero for me and catch the baby or cut the cord. Sitting by the head of the bed, holding my hand, and staying positive will be so much more helpful. I know you'll be great at that."

Another patient advised talking to your partner if you're fearful about permanently altering the way the he sees you sexually after he watches you deliver a baby. She told us, "I thought he would say, 'Well, then I just won't look.' But his response really surprised me. He said, 'This has nothing to do with our sex life. When I've seen you with the flu or hungover, that hasn't altered my ability to appreciate you when you're feeling and looking hot. This is just another one of those different situations—I can compartmentalize it." Remember that millions of couples have gone through the birth process and maintained their sexual relationship afterward.

Even if you discuss many of these issues in advance, you may both be surprised by how each of you reacts in the moment. Set guidelines and make your values clear, but try to be open about the unexpected. Just as it makes sense to have a plan B for your birthing plan, you should have a backup for your childbirth coach. No matter how well you plan everything out, there's no guarantee that your spouse or partner, family or friends, will be with you when you go into labor. If your partner is on a work trip in another time zone, or stuck in rush-hour traffic, you should have someone else on call to step in, even temporarily, until he is able to get to you.

Some women plan in advance for someone other than their partner to be the primary labor and delivery point person. If you or your partner have serious concerns about his ability to give you the physical or emotional support you need, now is the time to have the difficult conversation about choosing someone else to be by your side. And don't wait until the last minute to talk about this plan with your partner.

Since it won't be a decision you come to lightly, try to be as specific as possible with your concerns about why you think it's best for him to be number two rather than number one: You've seen him panic before when you've been sick, you're stressed by the way he talks to doctors, you're worried he might be so squeamish he'll faint. Or maybe you just want the pressure to be off him so he can experience childbirth without having to be in charge. Rather than excluding your partner, consider having him be part of a team alongside your mom, sister, friend, or doula.

As one of our patients explained, "I really wanted a doula— someone who knew what she was doing. My husband was a little insulted that I didn't think he'd be able to do it, but I explained that she would be there to support both of us, not to replace him. When the time came, she was able to teach him how to be helpful to me— they sort of worked together, and he felt like she was there for him, too. And he liked her even more when, hours into labor, she reassured him that nothing would be happening for the next few hours and forced him to go out and get something to eat so that he'd have more energy when it would really count."

If your partner is relieved that she doesn't have to play an active role, or if she's the one who raises the possibility of stepping back, you may feel hurt or like she's abandoning you. Remember, just because she doesn't match your idea of "perfect" in this circumstance doesn't mean she doesn't have other strengths or doesn't love you. You can acknowledge this limitation, and work on accepting it as a forgivable weakness, like the fact that she's a bad cook or is awkward at your office parties. It's important to remember that the day you give birth isn't necessarily a microcosm of your relationship, and it certainly can't predict how your partner will support you emotionally in the future.

If you're unpartnered, we highly recommend asking one or a few people to be on call for you when you go into labor. The benefits of choosing a family member (like a parent or sibling) are that you may feel like it's easier to let your most childlike needs out in front of them (because odds are, they have seen you in that state before). But if there's a friend who has already shown you through the pregnancy (and in life) that you can lean on her, she may feel like family or a partner already and will perfectly fit the bill.

In general, if you're asking someone other than your partner to be your labor go-to, don't forget to discuss the logistical details of being on call. If she's a single mother, who will watch her child if she has to come meet you in the middle of the night? Will your sister be able to leave work at a moment's notice if need be? Broach these questions well in advance, and offer help with finding solutions.

Other Family and Visitors

When you look beyond your one or two labor point people, you will also need to figure out who else (if anyone) is welcome in the delivery room and how you want to receive visitors after you've given birth. **We encourage you to be thoughtful, deliberate, and even self-centered as you set the rules.**

Some hospitals and birthing centers restrict the number of people allowed in the labor and delivery room. This can give you an easy out if your mother or mother-in-law wants to be in on the action and you don't want her there. It can also be a disappointment if you wanted her support. If you feel strongly about these policies, you can always talk to your doctor to learn more about why they exist and ask how your needs and concerns can be best accommodated.

Do not invite anyone to be present during your labor and delivery unless you're 100 percent sure you want her there, because if she gets in the way, you may not have the energy or clarity of focus to ask her to leave. No one should intrude on the privacy you deserve, even if she feels left out. That includes your mother and your partner's mother, or anyone you perceive as intimidating, critical, selfish, or demanding.

If you're giving birth at home or in a place where there are no restrictions on visitors, then you and your partner need to set your own limits. If you don't want your sister-in-law to let your child into the bedroom while you're in labor, say so. Make it clear that children can't come in, even if they're crying. Leave advance instructions to take them to the park, or a museum, or a movie, or consider finding someone your older child can stay with while you're in labor.

Some of us are more experienced with setting limits with family and have learned that those confrontations are often worth it. This is hard, and even more difficult if your past attempts to get space from your parents or in-laws have already been unsuccessful. One way to think about this issue is that there's going to be tension either way: If you're clear about your expectations on the front end, your family may be disppointed. But if you agree to arrangements that make you uncomfortable, you may become passive-aggressive, explosive, or regretful later.

As one patient explained, you can't always predict whom you'll upset, but if you can muster the courage to ask for what you want, your family may pleasantly surprise you: "My mom wanted to be in the delivery room, but I had to tell her that we wanted it to just be my husband and me. I felt bad—I'm her only daughter—but I'm glad I spoke up. She handled it much better than I expected, came into town the second day, and got to visit in the hospital and then be at home with us for the first few days, so I think it was great and special for all."

If you think that some family members may have the bad manners to insist upon an invitation to the delivery room, you have three options to regain control: 1) you can choose not to tell them you have gone into labor and notify them only after the baby is born; 2) you can give the hospital or birthing center strict instructions on whom to allow in; 3) your partner (or other designated person) can be assigned "birth bouncer" to make sure that no one uninvited barges in on you.

One of our patients told us she didn't invite anyone (other than her partner) to come to the hospital until after their son had been born. She felt like it was too much pressure to know that there were people in the waiting room just watching the clock. After the baby was born, her partner called her parents and in-laws, and they drove to the hospital to meet him.

Some families easily recognize that your birthing room is a private space that you control, but then they feel free to descend on you when and how they want to visit after the baby is born. It's important that you continue to set boundaries and make your expectations clear—in communication before and after your baby's birth. The intensity and vulnerability of delivery hardly disappear the moment your baby is born.

One patient struggled because she empathized with her husband's difficulty setting his own boundaries with his mother: "My husband's dad died when he was young, so he grew up with a single, widowed working mom. She sacrificed so much for him and had a hard time moving on after he grew up and moved out. I love how sensitive and caring he is about including her, so when she asked if she could fly in to be here for the baby's birth, he said yes, assuming that I would be as welcoming as always. But he didn't think about the details—she expected to stay at our place, as usual, and I ended up delivering a few days after my due date, so she was sleeping on our couch when I went into labor. I wish we'd talked through that before he decided."

Sometimes it's not easy to say no to family, especially to in-laws. Rather than set up the same fight with your partner about your in-laws that you've been having for years, we advise you to consider this as a new beginning and the perfect time to set some new boundaries.

You may want to designate someone to send out an announcement that you and the baby are doing well after the birth so that you don't have to be thinking about it or fielding questions when a savvy friend notices you haven't been online all day. This could be your partner, another family member, or a trusted friend. **Take your time to consider how much information you want to share and how to send out the news.** Pictures or no pictures? Social media post or group text? If you're open to friends visiting you in the hospital, do you want to specify "by invitation only" (so that those you invite don't spread it around to all your other relatives and show up with a giant entourage)? Do you want to say that all is well even if you had delivery complications? Or do you want to wait until you have a more complete sense of your or your baby's medical situation?

Consider whom you want to include on the list and whether they will all respect your wishes about visitors. Even if you draft your email list in advance, you may want to wait to compose the details about visiting invitations or privacy requests until the baby is here. Make sure your partner knows if you want a check-in before the announcement goes out. You can't anticipate how you'll feel after you deliver, and you may need and want time to recover without having to deal with company, even your immediate family.

Anyone invited to see you right after the baby is born should be someone with whom you feel comfortable under any circumstances. If you don't want to deal with the possibility of being seen in a postpartum diaper or with an exposed breast, or if they are going to question your decision to nurse or not nurse or otherwise make you feel criticized or stressed, they shouldn't be on the list.

In addition to spelling out whom you want to visit and when, you may want to think about certain guidelines for behavior. You can be clear with visitors if you don't want them to pick up the baby, to be in the room while you're nursing, to take photos, or to post on social media. One patient felt relieved by telling her partner in advance that she didn't want any photos taken of her: "I said that he could take pictures of the baby, but just my arms. I did not want to have to worry about looking like one of those glowing moms—I certainly wasn't going to bring any makeup or my blow-dryer to the hospital with me to give birth just for one of those stupid pictures. I wanted to focus on myself and the baby, not looking good for anyone else." If you can spend some time reimagining your birth experience, you may be able to better advocate for the boundaries that will make you feel most comfortable once the real day arrives.

A Hormonal Primer of Labor and Delivery

Hormones play a big role in how you experience childbirth, physically and psychologically—their ups and downs may take a toll on your mood, energy, cognition, and memory during and after the experience. Though every woman's specific physiology is different, the hormonal shifts during labor and delivery and immediately after may be the most dramatic of your entire life.

As we described in the hormone primer in Chapter One, your body's levels of **HCG, estrogen,** and **progesterone** rise during pregnancy. The signal for this escalation comes from the placenta. When the placenta is delivered after the baby is born, it's kind of like shutting off your hormonal faucet. As one of our patients described to us: "Over the next few days, I could feel my estrogen drop—and it felt like falling off a cliff. I felt my emotions become unstable, kind of like the worst PMS of my life. I wasn't exactly angry, just super-sensitive, like I had lost all the skin holding my feelings in and I was psychologically hanging out there, super-raw. If my mom looked only slightly unhappy, it made me super-irritable, and everything my sweet husband did made me cry like it was our wedding." In the **Appendix**, we'll explain how this hormonal crash causes the "baby blues" in most women; this temporary wave of emotional sensitivity and mood swings can last for up to two weeks. Knowing that it's coming—and that it's normal—can help you ride that initial wave.

There are other pregnancy hormones that help your brain and body prepare for childbirth and lactation. See below for a list of a few that have the strongest psychological effects:

Oxytocin. Before birth, oxytocin cues your uterus to contract, helping with the baby's passage through the birth canal (this is why the synthetic form of oxytocin, pitocin, is used by doctors to medically trigger labor). After birth, oxytocin helps to expel the placenta and close and heal your uterine blood vessels. Oxytocin also signals the "letdown reflex" that tells your breasts the baby will be here soon, so it's time to start making milk (suckling, or other forms of mechanically stimulating your nipples, may cause oxytocin to secrete). Oxytocin is often called the "bonding hormone" because it is associated with feelings of love, closeness, and a desire to protect.

Prolactin. This hormone is also secreted by your brain and, before pregnancy, is involved in your menstrual cycles. Like oxytocin, it generally rises during pregnancy and then surges during labor and after. Its main role is to signal milk production.

Endorphins. These hormones are sometimes referred to as the source of the "runner's high." In labor, they may be released by the brain as the body's natural painkiller and energy booster. (This could possibly explain why some women are able to stay awake and care for their babies after the exhaustion of childbirth.)

Epinephrine/norepinephrine. These are commonly called "stress hormones" and are released during labor and the body's fight-or-flight response to fear, which is naturally triggered by the intense pain of childbirth. They work to signal the body to do a variety of things to prepare for and recover from labor, and they may possibly contribute to a feeling of increased energy or anger.

Meeting Your Baby and Love at First Sight

Seeing and holding your baby for the first time is something most of us imagine as one of the most euphoric moments in life. The fantasy feeling of oneness that follows is perhaps at the core of what psychologically motivates many of us to become parents and, more specifically, to face the challenges of labor.

Some women do describe instantaneous, overwhelming feelings of awe, love, and connection with their new child. We've heard women say that the bond feels familiar, like they've been waiting all their life to meet this little person, and the fit feels just right, "a love I've never known possible" that washes over them when they first hold their baby. There's likely a biological basis to this sensation due to the oxytocin that surges immediately after delivering a baby and when a baby first suckles. And there is a biological foundation for an endorphin high that some women experience after delivery, filling them with extra energy so they may not feel tired until hours after birth. But even if every woman's body produces oxytocin and endorphins, not every woman's brain, nervous system, and psychology turn those hormonal signals into the same idyllic experience.

For the most part, love at first sight is a myth—whether on a first date or with a new baby. This doesn't mean you won't feel some intensity, but if you don't well up and feel an instantaneous surge, don't think there's something wrong with you. We've talked about the baby in your body; now you're meeting her for the first time. The relationship you had with the baby in your mind is different, and this new baby may not "feel" exactly like you imagined.

When first meeting your baby, you may barely be able to keep your eyes open due to exhaustion, or you may still be in pain. Especially if you've had a difficult delivery, you may feel relief more than anything else—relief that he's okay, that you're okay, and that labor is finally over. Or you may be focused on what's still happening in your body: delivering the placenta, stopping bleeding, or stitching up your C-section or episiotomy. As one patient described: "It was disappointing the first time I held my baby. I had a C-section and couldn't feel anything when he came out; I definitely didn't feel any emotional rush. All I could think was *Is he okay?* and *What is going on under that curtain with all that blood?* I couldn't enjoy anything in that cold operating room and couldn't wait to get out of there."

Many women who don't feel instant love for their baby may simply be taking time to grasp the massive shift in reality that's just taken place. Labor is usually a slow, gradual process, but the actual birth (when the baby is being pushed out of the vaginal canal or removed during a C-section) may happen at what feels like lightning speed. And in that instant, the energy in the room changes. Suddenly, *boom*, you and everyone in the room, no matter how many births they've seen, encounter the profound fact that something that began as DNA stardust is now in the world as a crying, suckling human being. As one of our patients put it: "I had this weird thought when I first saw him: *Who's that baby?* It took me quite awhile to recognize that he was truly mine. That I wasn't a pregnant woman anymore—suddenly, I was a mother."

If you're not able to focus on this first meeting, try not to feel upset with yourself, ashamed, or worried that you're not going to be able to love your baby. Yes, this is one of the most important moments of your life. But you're going to have a lifetime with your baby—you don't need to fit all your emotions into this single second.

Emotionally Processing Childbirth

You may have heard the folklore that women naturally forget their memories of childbirth, a bit of evolutionary engineering so they're not afraid to have more children. Some women agree that the psychological experience of childbirth is so intense, physically exhausting, and complicated by mind-altering medications and hormones that it's hard to remember the details. But it's a medical myth that your birth memories are evolutionarily programmed to fade. In fact, a fuzzy memory is just as common as a high-resolution one. Some women find that their memories of childbirth have a "halo effect," meaning that the positive feelings around meeting their baby overshadow any recollections of pain and fear. But others say that they remember every painful detail and find themselves replaying the worst parts for weeks.

Many women tell us that they are simply too busy after giving birth to reflect on what has just happened. There's so much to do: physically heal; learn how to care for your newborn; recover from the impact of hormonal shifts, medications, exhaustion, and pain; and deal with other family members and logistical concerns. One of our patients described it this way: "Even after I left the hospital, I needed to spend a lot of time—weeks, even (when I wasn't taking care of the baby)—looking out the window and spacing out before it occurred to me: *I just gave birth. That was crazy! What was it like again?* It was at least a month before I was able to think and talk about it."

If you're feeling odd about the fact that this amazing thing just happened to you and you haven't had any time or space to think about it, or you're just too tired to do so, trust that the experience will be there for you to process whenever you're ready. Don't feel burdened by having to understand anything you've gone through. Everyone metabolizes intense experiences differently. When you're ready, the very things you remember will be exactly what you need to process at that time.

How to Cope If Your Birth Experience Was Not What You Wanted

If your experience of labor and delivery did not match your idealized vision, you may feel like blaming your medical team, your partner, and/or yourself. Many of us have been influenced by social messages that some births are "better" or more "natural" than others. Yes, childbirth can be a celebration of a goddess-like capacity, but if your birth experience did not leave you feeling powerful, that's nothing to be ashamed of.

One patient shared this story: "I'm really connected to my body and its natural rhythms. One of my best friends is a doula, and we had been working together for months, preparing me mentally, physically, and spiritually for my home birth. But she also prepared me for the possibility that I might have to go to the hospital, and if that happened, it would be for the right, safe reasons. I labored for twenty-six hours at home—we used water, massage, breathing, stretching, aromatherapy, and herbs. The baby was just not advancing, and I was starting to get physically exhausted, like I really had nothing else to give. She and my midwife decided it was time to transfer me to the hospital, and I felt so ashamed, like I had failed them, my baby, and myself. Afterwards, I felt angry and cheated about my birth. But my midwife helped me stay focused on this: Sometimes birth just goes beyond our control, even when we do everything 'right.' I tried to repeat that to myself whenever I was feeling disappointed, and it helped to say the words. Then, one day, I really believed them."

If your child's birth wasn't what you'd hoped for—whether because of medical complications or a birth plan that got thrown out the window—it's not a referendum on your strength or mothering ability. And it's just one moment in a long childhood and even longer life. Attachment, bonding, your parenting dynamics, and your child's developmental narrative are experienced in a lifetime of moments, and this is just the beginning.

How to Recover from Birth Disappointment

If you're having a hard time letting go of upsetting feelings around your labor and delivery, here's some advice that may help:

- **Acknowledge the loss.** While you can and should forgive yourself and those around you for your labor's deviation from the plan, you may still have strong emotions about the gap between what you wanted and what you got. Facing these feelings may be the first step in the grieving process that will help you move on. You may also realize that you're actually upset about something deeper (for example, maybe your anger is not really about the C-section but about how your sister decided not to get on a plane in the middle of the night to be with you).

- **Talk about how you're feeling.** Confide in your partner, friends, or family members—anyone whom you can trust to listen without judgment and offer you support. Talk to other new mothers, too; you may be surprised to find out your experiences aren't as uncommon as you think.

- **Don't blame yourself.** What didn't go as planned wasn't your fault. If your delivery didn't go according to your birth plan, there may have been a good medical reason—asking your doctor to explain may help you appreciate that the change of plan was ultimately the healthiest choice for you and your baby. And if you made a choice you now regret in the depths of labor—for pain medication or intervention—again, don't blame yourself. Find compassion for the pain or fear you were feeling in the moment. If there was a medical complication like a premature birth, don't get sucked into thinking this was a consequence of anything you did wrong.

- **Ask for help.** If, after a few weeks, you aren't able to summon up positive feelings about your baby, and you still feel oppressed by negative thoughts, then it's time to talk to your caregiver about the possibility that you may be suffering from anxiety or postpartum depression. This may also be a sign that your delivery is stirring up some past trauma or was a traumatic experience on its own.

If You Had a Traumatic Delivery

If you feel that your birth experience was traumatic, then it was—simple as that. Some women have no trouble assimilating their childbirth experience into the narrative of their lives, even if they had a complicated or difficult birth. **But even a healthy birth can be triggering for trauma.** Women who have a history with hospitalization and medical procedures may run a higher risk of feeling traumatized. Furthermore, those who have experienced prior physical violence (sexual or physical assault) may feel particularly vulnerable and exposed during labor and delivery. Births with medical complications to the mother or child are also more likely to be experienced as emotionally traumatic.

Some of our patients who have been through traumatic birth experiences may fall into one of the following categories:

- **The Seal-overers.** For some of us, the first step to recovery is letting a wound scab over by moving on and doing things that distract us from our upsetting memories and make us feel calm and good. Yes, this is "denial," but as with pre-labor fears, denial can be a functional coping mechanism. If you force yourself to talk about a painful experience too soon, it can be "activating," stirring up disturbing feelings before you are ready to face them. If the most comfortable thing for you is not talking about those memories, then trust that instinct.

- **The Open-uppers.** If your strong feelings about your birth experience aren't fading, or you find yourself replaying your labor and delivery in your mind, voluntarily or not, don't ignore your feelings. Trying to do so may backfire; these memories and feelings may surface eventually, possibly in unproductive ways. Sometimes you can't avoid talking about an experience, and if this is happening to you, go with it. Don't be afraid to share your story with your partner, trusted friends or family, or in an online community. Journaling can also be helpful, as can talking to a therapist.

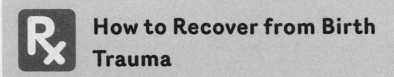

How to Recover from Birth Trauma

No matter what group you fall into, if you're feeling shaken or upset by your birth experience, consider these practical ways to help you cope:

- **Remember that perfect is the enemy of the good.** Don't judge your experience against that of other women, or against your previous experience if you have had other births.

- **Take control of the narrative.** Try reframing what happened to your body in the positive. Some women call the physical reminders of their birth experiences "battle scars" and consider them a sign of strength and resilience. Your body will heal, even if it takes more time than you thought; and remember the outcome of your wounds: your baby. If you're an open-upper, tell your story.

- **Heal from the outside in.** Take care of your post-labor body. You have to heal, and that healing will take rest and time. If you are in pain, tell your practitioner. Emotional pain can be caused or intensified by physical pain or injury (and vice versa.) It's not just that being in pain is upsetting—there's a physiological connection, too. The body's chemical response to physical damage, which includes inflammation, may be associated with the biology of depression. Other research shows that emotional stress can slow down the physical process of wound healing. If you're not sure what to do for your emotional self, taking care of your physical self is a powerful first step.

No matter how much self-help you employ, sometimes outside help is necessary. Women who struggle to process their birth experience may show signs of an acute stress reaction (if symptoms appear within four weeks after birth) or signs of post-traumatic stress disorder (PTSD) if symptoms last longer than four weeks. Symptoms of these conditions include:

- Nightmares and flashbacks
- Avoidance of anything that reminds you of the experience
- Extreme irritability
- Feeling isolated and isolating yourself from others
- Depression
- Being easily startled, trouble sleeping or concentrating, hypervigilance (being on guard)

People may develop PTSD when they or someone close to them have been through a life-threatening event. Not everyone who has a difficult labor or scary delivery will develop PTSD, but if you have a history of past trauma, or issues with anxiety or depression, you may be more susceptible.

PTSD requires assessment and treatment by a mental health professional, so if you're suffering from any of these symptoms, be sure to let your doctor know, and see our mental health **Resources**.

Pregnancy Loss

Sometimes labor and delivery doesn't have a good outcome. Whether problems were anticipated or unexpected doesn't make dealing with a devastating loss any less challenging. Entire books have been written on the subject, and it's beyond the scope of this one to address it with the care you deserve. The only thing we will say is that if this describes your situation, we hope that you use every support available to help you heal. You'll find more materials for pregnancy loss, stillbirth, and medical complications and conditions in our **Resources**.

The First Few Days After Birth

The first few days after delivery will be different depending on the circumstances of your birth: hospital vs. home, C-section vs. vaginal, medical complications for you or the baby vs. none. However, there are some common physical experiences of healing and early efforts to breastfeed (or deciding not to) that are emotional for most women.

Many women tell us how unprepared they were for what their bodies would go through in the first few days after delivery. Many women don't talk to each other about the graphic realities of their pregnant and postpartum bodies. We've heard different reasons for this ranging from "That's private" to "My friends wouldn't want to hear the gory details" to "It's gross" to "I've never heard of this before, so I must be in a freaky minority."

The cultural and psychological factors that lead women to be secretive about their sexuality and gynecologic health has been explored by scholars of history, politics, economics, religion, and anthropology. As psychiatrists, we are interested in the effects of these social stigmas; how keeping secrets about their bodies—and telling the truth—makes women feel.

What if social media helped women supportively talk to each other about their pregnant and postpartum bodies? As bad as social media can be for women's body image and self-esteem, it can also be a place where social norms about the female body can be disrupted.

One of our favorite examples of truth telling and the pregnant body is a Facebook post of a postpartum woman, her back turned, standing in the "diaper" she got in the hospital after delivery. (The "diaper" is absorbent underwear that works like a sanitary pad for the heavy flow of blood and fluids called "lochia," as well as urine, because bladder control may be difficult for some women.) Her husband is standing next to her holding their diapered baby, and everyone is laughing. In her post, the woman in the photo explains: "This is motherhood; it's raw, stunning, messy, and freaking hilarious all rolled into one. Having a baby is a beautiful experience, and the realities of postpartum life aren't spoken enough about."

Hundreds of thousands of women around the world were buzzing about this photo, sharing their own postpartum diaper stories, and tagging their pregnant friends on Facebook to let them in on the "secret." We think that this post went viral because women were sharing stories and giving each other advice about postpartum vaginal healing.

One woman reacted to the photo: "It's true, we don't talk enough about what happens in labor and delivery." Another woman added: "I can still feel the cold pack they put in that diaper that doubles as a giant pad down there—it helped me so much!" Another tagged her pregnant friend in a comment for the post: "Take some of these diapers home from the hospital—they're not easy to find and you're going to need them!"

As with any social media phenomenon, there were also naysayers, women who commented, "Is nothing private anymore?" Certainly, just as we have different personality styles, not all women want to be extroverted about this subject, and those people should feel comfortable unfollowing anyone whose posts are increasing their feelings of stress. Sometimes, taking a social media hiatus can be calming. Our hope, though, is that the women who do want to know "what to expect" can continue to be more open and less ashamed when talking about their pregnant and postpartum bodies in person and online.

Pain and Recovery

Even after an easy vaginal birth without any tearing or episiotomy, most women will experience physical discomfort after childbirth. While some people adamantly avoid all medications during pregnancy and breastfeeding, we encourage you to not fear using them as medically prescribed if you would benefit from some relief. As one of our patients suggested, "Don't be afraid to take the pain meds they offer. Your doctor isn't going to give you anything that's dangerous for the baby, and trust me, it will help you!" Rest and alternative and holistic approaches to postpartum pain management can be helpful, either instead of or in addition to medications—a postpartum doula should be able to assist you with these options. And of course, if you have concerns about which pain medications are associated with the risk of addiction, ask your doctor.

The First Few Days of Feeding

Whether you're adjusting to breastfeeding or deciding not to breastfeed, the first few days of feeding may be one of the most emotionally charged moments of the postpartum. We encourage you to read up on the physical advice for breastfeeding in books and on websites in our **Resources**. We're here to give you advice on the emotions of early breastfeeding.

In the last few decades, a breastfeeding advocacy movement has developed, pushing more lactation consultants into hospitals and promoting the many benefits of breastfeeding. These initiatives have helped many women, and many of our patients have told us they are grateful for that early support. Others have described breastfeeding as one of the most powerfully positive experiences in their parenting. For some the joy is emotional, and for others it leads to a physical sense of well-being and deep satisfaction.

The downside to this movement is that not all women can or want to breastfeed, and those women may face strong pushback for their situation or choice. Some of our patients have told us that feeding with formula has become stigmatized, and many women feel shamed for not breastfeeding, so much so that they may keep it a secret from other women. Women who are unable to breastfeed often ask us, "How come no one told me so many other women are unable or just don't do it?" We encourage women to speak more openly, because shame around not breastfeeding can trigger social isolation and other stressors that may be the tipping point toward postpartum depression.

As doctors, we think it's important to balance the education about all the benefits of breastfeeding with some of the benefits of *not* breastfeeding. We tell our patients "Fed is best," which means that adequate nutrition and hydration are more important than comparing breast milk and formula. While the American Academy of Pediatrics (AAP) promotes exclusive breastfeeding in the first six months of infancy, they do NOT discourage the use of formula. Let us repeat: formula is FINE. **Not breastfeeding is NOT equivalent to hurting or neglecting your baby in any way.** Formula is simply another way to give your baby food. If your baby is having difficulty suckling or you're having difficulty making enough milk, supplementing or feeding with formula may be the number-one healthiest choice for your baby.

Another benefit of not breastfeeding is that people other than you can feed the baby. (Pumping, which we'll discuss in **Chapter Six**, is another way to bottlefeed and get help from others.) This can give you more time to sleep, which can be essential for your physical and psychological health. It can give your partner more opportunity to bond with your baby—and your being well rested will likely improve your attachment experience with your baby, too.

Furthermore, women who do not breastfeed have more flexibility to return to taking preferred medications that may be important for their own health. We'll discuss breastfeeding and medications (including antidepressants) in full detail in the **Appendix**, but let this be a reminder that your and your baby's health are a complex inter-action of many, many factors, including nutrition, sleep, bonding, and psychological wellness. Feeding is just one piece of that picture.

The Secrets of Feeding

The following stories capture the range of advice that women have told us they wish they had known before their first few days of breastfeeding or formula feeding:

- **Breastfeeding is just as emotional as it is physical.** "I'm not sure I was aware of the emotions of breastfeeding—I just thought of it as a practical problem to be solved. I could really tell how the oxytocin was affecting me. I loved the feeling and sort of got addicted to it."

- **It might be painful.** "I hadn't known that breastfeeding was going to hurt in the beginning—*and* that the hurt would go away. It was hard and painful, but the best advice I got was to stick it out for a couple weeks, at least. I did, and it got better after about three weeks."

- **It might not happen right away; keep trying and asking for help. Also, be prepared with some formula even if your goal is exclusive breastfeeding.** "I had a beautiful home water birth, but nothing came out of my nipples for the first day, no matter all the tricks my doula tried. I didn't have any formula in the house because that absolutely was not my plan, and no one told me that we might need it for that kind of an emergency. When my baby was crying in hunger, I made my husband go out and get some formula. It took a few days, but my doula and I stuck with it and breastfeeding ended up working great for me. I loved it.'"

- **Do not equate breastfeeding with success and formula with failure.** "I wish I had allowed them to give him formula along with breast milk so we could have all relaxed about him getting enough food."

- **Every baby and every mom is unique when it comes to feeding.** "The best advice I ever got on breastfeeding was: Do as you feel is best for you, not what you think you should do."

- **If you don't want to pump, that's okay, too.** "I had an early delivery with twins and was running back and forth to the NICU while my C-section scar was still healing. Early on, I realized that pumping was just too much. The babies did great on formula, but I can't tell you how many times people asked me how breastfeeding was going. Why didn't people ask me how I was doing? People are so obsessed with breastfeeding, and I guess they're just trying to make conversation, but it felt really judgmental and exhausting every time I had to explain why I decided not to."

- **If breastfeeding experts give you conflicting advice, streamline your questions to your birth practitioner and pediatrician.** "I didn't like the hospital lactation consultant, who was bossy and seemed to give us advice that was conflicting with what the pediatrician said. I was, however, terrified, so whatever she told us to do, I did."

- **No matter how hard you try, it may be out of your control.** "For me, it was an issue that my baby wasn't able to latch. I tried all the tricks, but he did much better feeding from the bottle. I tried pumping, but my supply just wasn't enough. I was sad I couldn't breastfeed, but it was also a bit of a relief when we switched to formula—no more forcing something that doesn't work."

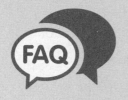

Labor and delivery are profoundly personal, so there's no way to capture every question we've been asked about the experience. The following are some of the most common:

Is it bad for bonding if I send the baby to sleep in the hospital nursery?

Many new moms fear that if they allow their child to sleep in the hospital nursery, it will interfere with the important early days of bonding and long-term attachment, or with breastfeeding. But ask a mom who is delivering her second or third child, and she will reassure you that your parenting style in the first few hours or days of your child's life—just like the rest of parenting—does not have to be heroic. And try not to think in terms of *should*, or what a "good mother" would do, but what you want and need in this moment. As one of our patients shared, "It's the only time you'll have a free baby nurse, so you'd be crazy not to take them up on it. If you're breastfeeding, you have to be up every three hours anyway, and you can just ask for them to bring him in and wake you up. If the baby is next to you, he's going to make noises, and you'll be worried about them and not sleep at all." Newborns spend most of their time sleeping, as their brains and bodies invest in a demanding growth spurt. Your baby is recovering from birth, too—he probably won't have the energy to be freaking out about your absence.

When your hospital nurse asks if you want to send your baby to the nursery while you sleep off your labor and delivery, we recommend you consider the option. Some things to think about if you're feeling guilty or worried about this decision:

- You need sleep to recover from childbirth.
- You should get rest now, because you won't get much at home.
- Hospital nurses are professional caretakers.
- You can always change your mind and ask that your baby return from the nursery after a few hours if you'd like (or vice versa).

Many women want to keep their babies in sight at all times because of catastrophic "what if" fears in the initial postpartum, such as: *What if my baby is kidnapped or switched and given to another family?* Even if you know these odds are low enough for this concern to be irrational, your fear is an understandable evolutionary response. We're hardwired to keep our children safe, and when you can't see your baby, an alarm bell may instinctually go off, putting you on guard for danger. If you notice yourself panicking from these sorts of worries, try to do some deep breathing. Also consider your level of exhaustion and physical pain, as this can sometimes trigger panic attacks. Once you're feeling calmer, it may help to reassess if it still feels best for you to keep your baby with you at all times rather than spend some time in the newborn nursery.

Of course, if it feels right to have your baby with you in the room, then follow that instinct and enjoy it. This desire is sometimes not about fear at all. You've never been physically separate from your baby, and it may feel right to stay physically connected on a primal level. It's also possible that your hospital nursery will not offer the option to keep a baby overnight.

How can I get emotional support if my baby has to go to the NICU?
Babies who are born prematurely and need monitoring or intervention may be brought to the hospital's neonatal intensive care unit, or NICU. Sometimes that stay is just for a night or two, and you'll be discharged to go home with your baby. Other times the stay is longer, and you may be making trips back to the hospital after you've been discharged.

While it can be heartbreaking and frightening when a baby needs medical attention, the NICU is absolutely the safest place for your baby to be. It may be helpful to think of the NICU as the best five-star treatment the hospital has to offer. The doctors and nurses who choose to work in the NICU have elected to get extra training because they love helping newborns. They're well versed in comforting babies in incubators, and they know how to deal with the most challenging of medical issues.

If your baby is in the NICU longer than a day or two, you may worry that you won't be able to bond with her. **It may also feel very wrong that you're not able to hold her, or bring her home with you.** It is natural to feel anxious, even panicky, about this separation.

Know that there are ways you can bond with your baby while he is in a NICU incubator or connected to monitors and tubes. Even very premature babies can benefit from "kangaroo care," where a baby is taken out of the incubator and placed on his parent's chest for skin-to-skin bonding. Most hospitals will encourage this if your baby is medically stable, because it can decrease parents' anxiety and has benefits for the baby.

If your baby is not medically allowed out of the incubator, he may still be able to benefit from therapeutic touch: You don't need to hold your baby for him to feel your presence and to begin to create the bonds of attachment. Cradling his head in your palm can soothe him; the NICU nurses can show you how. They can also show you the signs that he's enjoying the contact. You can take pride in the care you're giving him and the beginning of your bond.

Each NICU has different rules about when and how often parents or others can visit. If you want to spend more time with your baby, or to participate more actively in her care (and it's medically safe to do so), advocate for yourself and your partner. But also remember to take care of yourself. Some moms don't give themselves permission to leave the NICU because they believe that their presence protects their baby. It's important to remember that there are doctors and nurses caring for your baby 24/7, and that postpartum healing requires you to sleep.

Even if you know that your baby is getting the best care, most parents feel upset about the need for medical monitoring. Our patients have told us how hard it was to miss that first skin-to-skin contact (if their baby is in an incubator and not ready to be held for long periods of time) or not be able to breastfeed their babies (some premature babies need to be fed slowly through tubes before they're ready to suckle).

We encourage you not to push down your feelings of disappointment, grief, loss, or anger. One supportive feature of many NICUs is that they may have staff social workers available to sit down and talk about both logistics and how you're feeling. Like the NICU nurses, these social workers are trained in helping you with any and all emotional responses—so feel free to let out your tears, your rage, and anything that feels cathartic. Also consider support groups or online communities (see **Resources**).

If you're being pulled down further into sadness or distress about your baby, here are a few tips to help you gain perspective:

- Your immediate postpartum hormones may be making you feel more emotionally sensitive than usual.

- This experience is likely to be temporary. Just because you and your baby aren't having the immediate postpartum experience at home that you wanted doesn't mean that you won't be able to have it eventually, when your baby is discharged.

- When you're ready to see it, if you look around the NICU, you may be able to appreciate what a special place it is. As one mom explained, "My second child had to go to the NICU for prematurity, so I could compare it to the experience of going home right away with my first. Sure, I wasn't happy that she came early, but it really was so much easier than with my first. I was able to heal from my C-section and knew that the baby was in great hands. The NICU nurses are so patient and taught me again how to give a newborn a bath and tie a swaddle, and even called in a free lactation consultant to help me with breastfeeding issues. By the time my daughter came home, I felt ready for her. I hate to admit it, but I even miss the NICU sometimes because it felt so safe and supportive for both of us."

- The NICU is a community of new parents going through similar experiences, other mothers and fathers who can be a source of support and advice. We've heard many stories of women who met each other in the NICU and bonded during the hours sitting with their babies, side by side in hospital chairs, later becoming close friends and celebrating their children's birthdays together.

- If you want to breastfeed, but your baby isn't ready or medically cleared, start pumping. That will keep your supply flowing and give you the opportunity to feed your baby pumped milk through medical tubes and eventually a bottle. Remind yourself that you'll be able to try breastfeeding later, and in the meantime, you can stock up on a helpful supply of frozen milk to use down the road when you're sleeping or at work.

- As with other medical issues in pregnancy and pediatrics, try not to google statistics about your baby's diagnosis or day-to-day medical results. You won't find anything on the internet that's tailored to your baby's circumstances, so it's easy to get spooked by fears that have nothing to do with your baby's actual prognosis. Rather than going to the internet, we encourage you to keep a detailed list of questions and work with the doctors and nurses to get answers.

Why am I so anxious about circumcision?

Circumcision, or the removal of a male baby's foreskin, is part of some religions and cultures. It is also culturally common in the United States, and it may be offered as a procedure for your son before he leaves the hospital. Some pediatricians and ob-gyns recommend circumcision for health and hygienic reasons, though others debate these benefits.

Some parents don't even question whether they'll circumcise their babies, and others are unsure or second-guess their plan when the time comes. If that happens to you, don't pressure yourself to make the decision immediately—circumcision does not have to be done before leaving the hospital.

There are arguments on both sides, for and against circumcision, and we encourage you to do as much research as feels right for you. **But know that, as with so many other parenting decisions, this isn't a test you'll pass or fail.** Your partner may have strong feelings, connected to his own circumcision or lack thereof. It's impossible to say how your child will feel in the future about your decision, but as parents, you can do your best to help him grow up accepting his body as it is, whatever that looks like. You can talk to trusted friends, your pediatrician, and your religious leaders about the risks and benefits and how other parents face the same issues you're considering.

If you decide to move forward with circumcision, for religious or other reasons, you may be worried about your son being harmed by this minor surgical procedure. As with any other intervention with your child, you should research who is doing the circumcision and demand the doctor spend as much time as is necessary to explain the procedure and answer any questions you may have. Ask them about their statistics of outcomes—since this is a simple and straightforward procedure, most pediatricians and practitioners will have reassuring information.

Another common area of concern is that your baby will be in pain. Even if you know that the procedure is minor, it's not unusual to feel guilty about electing surgery that will cause your baby discomfort. Many parents think, *Why do I need to put him through this when he's so little?* Or: *I already cringe when I hear my baby cry. I can't stand to think that he'll be crying in pain.* These are reasonable responses that you should include in making your decision, but if you know intellectually that you want your son to be circumcised, it may continue to feel like the right decision for you.

Circumcision may be the first medical intervention you'll encounter with your baby. If your only hesitation is fear of inflicting pain on your baby, consider that at some point soon (nail cutting or, later, vaccinations) you'll have to participate in some activity that causes your baby discomfort but is ultimately in his best interest. The feeling of hearing him cry may get easier, or it may remain exquisitely painful—either way, you'll have to learn how to get through it.

We could write a whole book on this topic of labor and delivery, but since we have only one chapter, we encourage you to review our **Resources**, which go into more detail about the physical recovery from childbirth and have been shaped by medical practitioners and doula and midwife experts who spend the most time in the trenches with women during childbirth.

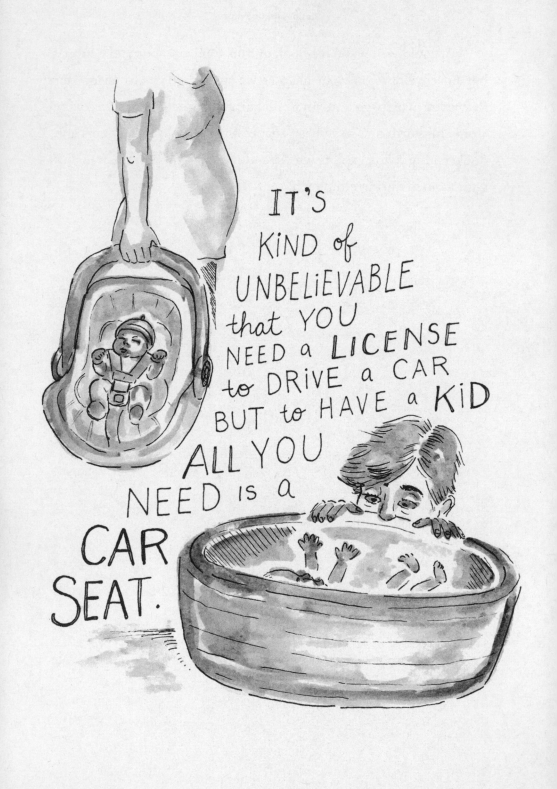

The Fourth Trimester

Coming Home to Your New Life

The first three months of your baby's life are unofficially called "the fourth trimester." If every trimester of pregnancy documents your baby's development, then you can think of the fourth trimester as the remaining months after birth when your baby continues to rapidly grow in his body, brain, and cognitive capacity. Since newborns behave similarly to how they did in the womb—mostly eating and sleeping—and are not yet dynamically interactive, many people think of the fourth trimester as an extension of fetal life. But calling this time the fourth trimester reveals how baby-centered our culture is, and obscures the fact that it's not at all a continuation of pregnancy for you—this is your *first* trimester of motherhood, a radically new phase in your life.

The fourth trimester marks a new phase in your matrescence. You got through pregnancy, and you got through childbirth. And look what you created: this tiny, beautiful human! This person who didn't exist before is now here, and not only does his heart know how to beat on its own, he already knows how to grab your finger and drink milk, just because nature intended it to be that way. It's sci-fi and it's thrilling. This is your first day at home together, and you're the mother. The feeling is sweet, shocking, and scary all at once.

But just as you've started to enjoy the peace and quiet, it will probably be pierced by the baby's cry, or a silence that may jolt you awake from your first few hours of sleep with a terrifying thought: *WHAT HAPPENED? WHERE'S THE BABY?* Multiple times a day you may ask yourself, *Am I doing this right?* and wonder, *Where are the real grown-ups? What are they thinking, leaving me alone with this child?* One of our patients put it this way: "It's kind of unbelievable that you need a license to drive a car but not to have a kid—all you need is a car seat."

One of the biggest adjustments to new parenthood is to the new level of uncertainty in your life. When you were pregnant, you walked around with your baby safely nestled inside your body. After birth, your baby becomes a physically separate being, and carrying him outside your body requires an entirely new set of psychological, physical, and cognitive skills. Yes, you're his mother, but that doesn't mean you'll intuitively know how to take care of him.

Even as you gain expertise and comfort, nothing will be predictable. Just when you're feeling like you have a routine, the baby will have a growth spurt with a change in her behavior and needs, and you'll be back to square one. As with other new experiences, it's natural to feel like you're *not* on top of it—the first time your baby falls asleep in your arms . . . and also the first time her diaper leaks and stains your rug.

Newborns' fragility adds to the high stakes—and frayed nerves—of early parenting. As one of our patients shared: "I thought the first bath would be so sweet, but instead, I was so afraid of him drowning—he was suddenly slippery. I didn't enjoy it because I was holding on to him so carefully, and then I worried I was squeezing him too hard—then I worried I could crush him. It's like the feeling I get when I'm traveling and have to take out my passport—that sudden fear: *What if I lost it?* When you know that something risky is possible, you see it flash before your eyes—the responsibility is overwhelming."

We hear worries like hers from almost every new parent: *How do I know the baby will keep breathing while we both sleep? How do I know if I'm feeding her enough? Is it dangerous if she throws up? Is his neck going to be permanently damaged if I forget to support his head and it flops forward or back?* These questions are always appropriate to bring to your pediatrician or partner, friend, or relative for reassurance. You'll learn how common it is to worry and rare it is for these worst fears to come true.

You are evolutionarily programmed to keep your baby alive—
and the younger and more fragile your baby is, the louder your
innate alerts will be. But just because your gut is telling you to be
ON GUARD, that doesn't necessarily mean that your baby is in any
danger—it usually just means that you're being attentive and careful.
But, hour after hour, this experience of being ALERT and ON can
be exhausting and, for many new parents, anxiety-provoking.

Anxiety isn't always a psychiatric symptom—it's also a healthy
human response to times when we need to pay attention and be
careful. You should be alert when you're driving so that you can avoid
an accident. The same is true when taking care of a newborn. The
good news is that both cars and infants are designed to withstand
imperfections from their caretakers.

As fragile as they seem, babies are remarkably resilient; they have
survived all sorts of unruly conditions without medical-grade care
for millennia. Even today, there are families raising perfectly healthy,
happy children in homes without electricity, let alone a baby monitor. Even when you feel frazzled and out of control, remind yourself
that your baby is designed to withstand the care of a human—that
means imperfect—mother.

Mindful Meditation for the Fourth Trimester

Sometimes the best way to calm down when your mind is rattling with worries is to simply let go, accepting the fact that you're worried instead of fighting it. Mindful meditation can be helpful to build as a daily practice, so that you can live with troubling thoughts but experience them with less emotional suffering. Meditation isn't inherently religious or spiritual—it's simply about noticing your thoughts and developing an ability to accept them so that they are less agitating. Meditation can help to detach those thoughts from their psychological power. There are many different schools of meditation; please see our **Resources** for some options. The following are some good ways to start:

- **Ten minutes a day.** As variable as your routine may be, setting up some regular rituals for yourself during these first few months can be a calming reminder that there's still some order in your universe. Pick one time in the day when you think you'll be able to stay awake while your baby is napping or being cared for by your partner. Find a sturdy chair and sit comfortably with your feet flat on the ground and your back straight, or if you're comfortable, sit upright on the floor. Set a timer for ten minutes,

close your eyes, and do your best to just sit there and breathe. It may help to start by counting your breaths, slowly inhaling through your nose and exhaling through your mouth. Once you count ten breaths, come back to one. If you notice that your mind has wandered off from the counting, don't feel bad—wandering is what minds do. Just notice that it happened, and come back to counting. Do your best to do nothing and observe without judgment: How does your body feel? What thoughts are bubbling up in your mind? You'll probably think of a flood of tasks you have to do. Don't stop to write them down. Just notice them, as if you're watching the landscape from a train window and the thoughts are passing by. Trust that you'll remember the important things later.

- **Body scan.** Take a few deep breaths, noticing how the breath feels while entering and exiting your body. Then take a mental tour of your body, noting any feelings or sensations as you go. Start with your head, then move down your neck to your shoulders, arms, torso, pelvis, legs, and feet. Go slowly—noting any tensions, the touch of clothing on your skin, whether you feel warm or cold—and with as much focus as you can, as if your awareness is a tiny point traveling through your body. If you get distracted, notice and accept it—you can even think, *I got distracted*—and pick up where you left off.

- **Moving meditation.** If you find that sitting still is too hard (or too difficult to stay awake), try a moving meditation. You can do this with any activity that doesn't require too much thinking and effort, like going for a walk, eating a meal, soaking in the tub, doing some stretches or yoga, or playing with or feeding your baby.

  In a moving meditation, your eyes are open, and your goal is to be curious about all of your senses. If you're feeding, look at your baby, your body, and the room as if you've never seen anything like this before: What does the baby's chin look like? What does the fuzz on his head look like? What about the shadows or light in the room? What about your own nails and hand? If a critical thought (*You really should get a manicure*) pops up, try to let it pass like a cloud through a clear sky. You can try the same thing with eating (pretend this is the first bowl of pasta of your life: How does it taste and smell? What does the texture feel like on your tongue?), touch (try washing your own skin in the shower as if you're blind and discovering the contours of a new body), and sound (even a sound as grating as your baby's cry can be interesting if you pretend you're a Martian and you've never met a baby before). As strange as this exercise may initially feel, allowing yourself to focus on your senses without judgment is a proven way to stay emotionally present and let go of your worries about the past and future.

One of the greatest regrets we hear from mothers looking back on the first few months with their babies is they were so preoccupied with their goals and plans that they missed the opportunity to enjoy this very short phase of their baby's life. As one of our patients described: "I wish I had taken more time to sit with my baby and just enjoy him." Another patient who is a mother of three shared this wisdom: "I know how quickly this newborn phase passes, and this is my last baby for sure, so I'm trying not to beat myself up for being such a mess. I am trying to be less strict with myself. I am trying to be more present." Mindfulness is the art of being present; if you practice ten minutes a day, you'll get hours of memories back in return.

Beginning One Marathon While Recovering from Another

Whether you delivered vaginally or had a C-section, your body has just gone through a major ordeal. Traditionally, your doctor or midwife may have given you some general instructions, like not exercising or having sex for a while, and how to care for any stitches or healing incisions you may have. But if you aren't scheduled to have a follow-up appointment for six weeks or more after delivery, this is a shockingly long time to be off on your own, especially since your doctor probably wanted to see you often during your pregnancy. As much as you may have complained about having to go to the doctor before, if she is not requesting to see you in the first few weeks after childbirth, you may feel abandoned and neglected. It may also reinforce the message you'll be getting from many sides: The baby's care is more important than yours.

If you'd just come out of the hospital after a different surgery, no one would expect you to manage on your own without a checkup for over a month. Thankfully, in 2018 the American College of Obstetrics and Gynecology (ACOG) came out with new guidelines for doctors to schedule the postpartum appointment at three weeks after childbirth; hopefully, common practice will follow these recommendations so that women will receive better care in the first few weeks of the postpartum period.

Expecting yourself to seamlessly pivot to caring for a newborn after the physical and emotional demands of birth is unrealistic. Many women have a hard time reconciling the fact that even if they feel energized to hit the ground running in new motherhood, their bodies just aren't keeping up. **How can you take care of a newborn if you can barely walk?** Because new moms aren't taught to focus on their own healing during this time, many criticize themselves for being lazy or selfish if they drag their feet when the baby cries.

In some cultures, family or neighbors step in to help a new mother recover from childbirth. In China, this period of time is called *zuo yue zi*, or "sitting the month." The focus is on the mother's healing: Relatives cook nurturing food and help manage the household. Typically, American society doesn't provide that kind of support, in either an intergenerational, communal, or public way.

It's not only that American culture doesn't have the expectation of family support for a new mother—it's sometimes logistically impossible. When Americans leave their extended families to work in bigger cities, about a quarter of them are no longer within driving distance of family members who might have otherwise helped with a new baby. This means increased stress, isolation, and expense for the new parents.

In many other countries, when families are not able to step in to help with child care, there is a social structure for support. In France, the government subsidizes day care AND pelvic floor physiotherapy (to help with pelvic and vaginal recovery); in Sweden, you get over a year of paid leave, and paternity leave is common; in New Zealand, new mothers can get a postpartum visit in their own home to check in on their physical and emotional well-being. None of these services is similarly subsidized in the U.S. And since there aren't laws in the U.S. that guarantee paid leave for fathers and grandparents, even if your partner and parents are local and willing, they may not be able to take time off from work to help you. No wonder the average American new mother feels so overwhelmed.

We say this not to be pessimistic but to encourage you to seek out help and create support systems however you can, and to reassure you that needing help is normal. Even if you prided yourself on your independence before, now is the time to call for backup. You may have envisioned these first weeks of parenthood as an intimate time for bonding as a new family; if you need some extra helping hands in the beginning, you'll still get plenty of quiet time later. Maybe you can ask family members to use a few vacation days to help out for a bit—you might be surprised by their willingness. Or, if you can afford it, hire a child care professional. If you don't have any references, call your hospital or birthing center, or ask your provider, doula, or friends for recommendations, and see our **Resources.**

Whether you have help with child care or not, you'll have to figure out how to make some time to care for yourself. Self-care is not selfish—it's self-preserving. One of the hardest parts of new motherhood is making time for activities that may sound frivolous but are actually essential to your sense of self. These are the experiences that make *you feel like you.*

Make a To-Do List for Your Self-Care

Sometimes the most identity-affirming activities are not obvious to us until we stop doing them. When we stop our usual routines, it's easy to feel disconnected from ourselves without knowing exactly why. Though it may sound obvious, depriving yourself of all the small things that give you daily pleasure can lead to feelings of depression.

We suggest that you make a list of your self-care essentials and put a copy of the list where you will see it several times during the day, like the bathroom mirror and/or the refrigerator door, to remind yourself to make space for those habits. Think about your life before the baby. What were the most physically *and emotionally* essential parts of your day? Or, in a given week, what were your favorite pick-me-ups? It can be helpful to brainstorm by category, from the small and essential to the large and indulgent. This list covers some examples, but we encourage you to be as detailed and eccentric as you can about the habits and activities that make you feel better:

- **Body:** Go to the bathroom, drink water, sleep, eat, shower (or at least wash your face and comb your hair), brush your teeth, exercise (when you're ready), go outside, put on clean clothes, get a haircut, return to your normal grooming.
- **Social/spiritual:** Texting or meeting up with friends, talking to family on the phone, volunteering, going to your house of worship, salsa dancing, gardening, meditating, taking a bath, getting a massage, watching TV, listening to music, playing an instrument, journaling, window-shopping, cooking or eating a delicious meal, spending time with people in whom you can really confide and who can remind you to laugh.
- **Relationship:** Date nights, sex (when you're ready), cuddling, talking to each other about your day, watching TV together, socializing with friends as a couple, resuming something pleasurable from your old routine like going out for a walk together.
- **Intellectual:** Reading a book, catching up with the news, going to the movies, visiting a museum, seeing a play, doing the crossword

puzzle, writing, talking to a colleague about work, talking to a friend who is interesting (consider if it would feel refreshing to steer clear of kid-related conversations).

Don't worry about the feasibility—brainstorm the list. If something seems unrealistic, consider how you can modify for your motherhood life—if you can't take a thirty-minute bath, can you soak your feet in the tub for ten minutes? If you can't afford to go out to dinner, can you ask someone to cook you a meal? This is an important practice to start now. If you tell yourself, *I'll get to that when the baby is older,* decades may pass before you happen to find the time. It may help to schedule personal appointments like haircuts or visits with friends the way you do a pediatrician's visit: at the end of the last appointment. Once it's on the calendar, you're more likely to remember your own needs and actually go.

The Fourth Trimester

Imagine what it's like to enter the outside world after living in the womb, where you're always warm, swaddled by the sides of your mother's body, and comforted by her heartbeat. No matter how cozy the nursery, it's a downgrade.

Even if she's born full-term, a newborn baby has years of

development to go through before she can function easily in the world, let alone take care of herself. One study showed that a human baby would need to undergo a gestation of over eighteen months (instead of the usual nine) to be born as neurologically and cognitively developed as a newborn chimpanzee. Humans deliver our babies very early in their development, and scientists aren't sure exactly why. The long-standing theory is that the human pelvis needs to be relatively small so that we can walk upright, which is at odds with the size of an older baby's head, which passes through the pelvis in childbirth. An eighteen-month-old baby may be more appropriately developed for survival, but that head would never fit through a mother's hips. Newer theories about the nine-month cutoff also have to do with metabolic competition between mother and fetus—essentially, that's the point when a developing fetus needs more of a mother's calories than she can safely provide before the relationship becomes dangerously parasitic.

Whatever the evolutionary reason, your baby arrives after nine months, extremely needy and somewhat half-baked. For the first few weeks especially, he barely fits the image of an adorable baby, and he's not much fun to be around. He may be sleepy and disengaged because his brain and sensory abilities are still developing. Plus, he's spending most of his energy growing, recovering, and adapting to this new environment we call planet Earth.

On the one hand, it's a blessing, because your newborn may sleep sixteen hours a day—although far from in one stretch—and he doesn't need as much stimulation as an older baby. But that's not to say newborns are easy. They still demand constant attention, and many moms say it's hard to feel attached to a creature who looks and acts like a blob from outer space. Newborns are often scrawny and wrinkled and nowhere near as cute as they will be when they plump up in a few weeks or start smiling and interacting with you in a few months. It will be that smile that gives you the feeling "She loves me! I'm her mama! Taking care of her is rewarding!" Until then, you may not be feeling so warm and fuzzy—especially not at four a.m.

Particularly if this is your first baby, it's natural to be concerned that feeling bored around your baby will last forever. But we've seen again and again that for many mothers, when their child gets older, bigger, a little bit more predictable, and a lot more communicative, caretaking becomes more fun.

One of our patients shared this story and the advice that worked for her: "During the first four weeks, every day felt the same, and I didn't feel any reward or connection for a while. It helped me to remember that at this stage, my baby was more of an animal than a real person: She eats, sleeps, and poops. If you want to watch TV while you're breastfeeding, don't feel guilty about that. She's getting what she needs from your body."

The Good Enough Mother

One of the most powerful ideas in the psychology of motherhood came over half a century ago, in the 1950s, when psychoanalyst Donald Winnicott coined the phrase "the good enough mother" in his writing and research. Winnicott saw that aiming to be a perfect mother is not only unnecessary but harmful. You don't need to be "the best" mother in order to raise your child well. You simply need to be good enough.

Some women think that good enough is not acceptable because it sounds like settling. They're working hard at the job of mother-hood and have made sacrifices, so shouldn't the results be better than just good enough?

Winnicott's idea is less about aiming for a low bar and more about accepting this fact: You can only do your best.

A marker of psychological wellness is being able to accept that no one is perfect. Even if your child is perfect in your eyes, he's also human. He may be a bad sleeper or a picky eater. He may grow up to struggle in school or fail at his chosen career. The sooner you accept that you're not going to be a perfect mother, the sooner you can start to prepare yourself that your baby is not going to be perfect, either. Rather than trying to achieve the goal of being a flawless mother, aim for compassion and authenticity when you're with your baby. That imperfect parent is the person your baby is going to love, and the model that your child will learn from as he grows up.

Since you are bringing your baby into an imperfect world, it's actually a pretty useful parenting trick to accept that you are flawed, too. If you were perfect and your child got used to that, he would never be able to hack it in the real world. Your job is to ensure that your child becomes an independent person, and if you're perfectly meeting his every need and want, that won't happen.

An imperfect mother helps her child gain the skills to tolerate frustration, become self-sufficient, and learn to soothe himself. These are necessary foundational skills for developing resilience, the ability to weather an emotional storm, and grit, the ability to persevere and achieve.

Ambivalence: The Push and Pull of Motherhood

We often hear moms whisper in hushed tones something they'd never tell their friends or partner: "Sometimes I wish I had my old life back." Or they wonder, *Am I a bad mother because sometimes I'd rather take a nap than nurse my baby?* These ambivalent thoughts are completely natural, yet many moms feel ashamed of them.

We call this the push and pull of motherhood—sometimes you'll feel pulled toward your baby's needs and your identity as a mother, and sometimes you'll want to push it all away. **Motherhood, like all complex experiences in life, is a mix of both positive and negative.** Loving your child doesn't change the fact that sometimes the work of caretaking is not fun. Yet for many moms, admitting that there are moments, days, or even weeks when you want a break from your baby is scary because it can make you ask yourself: *Am I trapped with this feeling forever? What if I made a mistake? Does this mean I don't love my baby?*

Feelings of ambivalence come up when you find that your attention is being pushed away from your baby to care for yourself and other people in your life, and you're not sure how to make that work.

Every time you make a choice, someone gets shortchanged. How are you not going to feel guilty about leaving a meeting at work to go to the pediatrician? Or sleeping an extra fifteen minutes while your baby is fussing, only to find him lying in spit-up when you go to fetch him? And what about when you're spending time with the baby but you're thinking about returning your friend's call, replying to your boss's email, eating dinner with your partner, or sleeping?

It's not always a bad thing to feel guilty. Guilt, like ambivalence and worry, may be an inherent state of motherhood. Sometimes guilt comes from comparing yourself to an unrealistic ideal. But other times guilt is a clue that you should reassess your choices. It can be productive if it encourages you to reflect on your actions and make any necessary changes. If you feel guilty because you're consistently late when you pick up your daughter from day care, for example, it may be time to sit down with your boss and discuss a formal change to your schedule, or find someone else to pick her up.

While guilt may be inevitable and often instructive, shame is a different thing. Guilt is feeling bad about something you did. Shame, on the other hand, is feeling bad about who you are as a person. Shame is concluding, *I'm bad at this and don't have what it takes to be a good mother.* Shame can make you feel trapped and desperate, so you isolate yourself from the support of other moms who—unbeknownst to you—are probably sharing many of the same experiences.

Different people may react to the same experience with shame or with guilt. One mother might feel a twinge of guilt for spending time on the phone while she's with the baby; accordingly, she may commit to putting the phone away and making more of an effort tomorrow, or she may decide that even though her choice is imperfect, it's working for her. Another mother might feel ashamed because she thinks that looking at her phone means that she doesn't love her child enough and that there's something wrong with her.

Shame is painful and sometimes irrational. And shame may lead to self-hatred, which may contribute to depression. Depression may make you want to be alone, which further cuts you off from sharing your feelings with others. When you're isolated from others, your sense of shame may be amplified, and the cycle continues, less a circle than a miserable spiral. People who are ashamed try to cover up what they're ashamed of. They don't talk about what they're feeling. Their buried feelings feed their self-hatred, and so on. Whenever you identify that you're feeling shame, the first step is to remember that feeling bad about an experience does not make you a bad person. Life is all about learning from our experiences: You can always choose differently next time.

Reframing Shameful Thoughts

When you feel shame, you can reframe what you're feeling with one of these more positive alternatives: **accomplishment** (rather than focusing on how you're failing, remind yourself what you're doing well); **gratitude** (instead of pointing out what's missing, pay attention to all that you have right now); **acceptance** (instead of raising the bar to be a "better mother," accept how much is out of your control, and that your goal should be "good enough" under those circumstances).

1. **Shameful voice:** "I am totally 'leaning out.' All of my friends are advancing at work—I had planned to update my CV while I was on maternity leave, and I haven't even turned on my computer. I guess I'm just lazy."

   Accomplishment reframe: "I have done a great job taking care of my baby and a pretty good job taking care of myself during maternity leave. It's an accomplishment that I have a job, and when I'm back at work, I'll prioritize what's next for me professionally."

2. **Shameful voice:** "I'm a bad mom already—it's horrible that I'm fighting with my partner about who is going to watch our daughter so I can go to my exercise class. I'm pathetic for being so

selfish, and for gaining all this weight anyway, which is why I'm so desperate to get to the gym."

Gratitude reframe: "It's okay that my partner and I are still figuring things out with our time management as new parents. I'm lucky to have a supportive partner who doesn't hold grudges after our fights. I'm glad I'm motivated to exercise, and I'm also lucky that my body is strong and healthy—this extra weight is how I was able to have a baby, and there's nothing wrong with my body as it is."

3. **Shameful voice:** "It's terrible that I put the TV on when I'm nursing. Why am I not more focused on loving my daughter when I'm nursing? I'm a terrible mother."

Acceptance reframe: "I'm with my daughter, actively engaging, most hours of the day. Breastfeeding has been stressful for me, and there's nothing I can do to fix that. If TV is what I need to help distract me so that I can get through a feed, and the baby's not staring at it, then what is so bad about that? And even if I am not so great at breastfeeding, that doesn't mean I'm a bad person or a bad mother. "

To survive as a mother-baby unit, you'll have to learn to live with the emotional tension created by this push-and-pull dance of caring for self and others. Shifting between seemingly contradictory feelings can make you feel like you don't know where you are emotionally, but neither feeling negates the other. It's the normal waves of motherhood.

Where Did the Day Go?

No matter how much you love your baby, there may be times when you feel like you're her servant. Ironically, this entry into parenthood may, even subconsciously, remind you of the powerlessness of your own childhood. You're not wrong—for a while, you have lost some control of your time management. Most new mothers we know have said to us, "I don't know where the day goes."

Many of our patients have unrealistic expectations about what they will be able to accomplish during a day when they're taking care of their newborn. Some women think that motherhood will be the start of a new, super-efficient phase of their life, going to the gym at five a.m. before the baby wakes up, or sending every thank-you note within twenty-four hours of receiving a gift. Others expect to be able to continue their pre-baby routine, getting work done while the baby sleeps or running errands with an infant strapped to their chest.

In our experience, the higher the bar you set, the easier it is to feel like you're failing yourself when you can't reach it. Unlike other times in life, when goals can be motivating, the first weeks with a newborn are a time when almost everything is out of your control. If you make lofty plans in the morning and then berate yourself at night for not living up to them, you'll just end up in a power struggle with yourself. You may also set up a power struggle with your baby if you try to force him into a strict schedule that he may not be developmentally ready for.

When moms hold tight to an idealized vision of what they can accomplish in a day, they may project their disappointment in and anger at themselves onto their babies. One patient said that she yelled at her baby for throwing up right after they left the house because "we didn't have time to go back home and start all over again." But when she caught herself blaming her baby for, well, being a baby, she not only felt disappointed for the hours lost, she felt guilty for her own misdirected frustration. The best advice to help her was simply to surrender to the experience. She learned to make plans that could be changed or broken, and to remind herself that this feeling of timelessness and chaos was temporary and would change in a few months, when her baby would be older and more able to settle into a routine.

Mastery is the feeling of having accomplished something, of knowing what you're doing and doing it well, and it's an important component of self-esteem. But caring for a baby is the opposite of mastery. There's no sense of accomplishment to be found when every clean onesie gets dirty within a few minutes, or when a fed baby is hungry again in two hours. **We recommend that you look for small, discrete tasks that you can accomplish to completion with little struggle.** Think small: clearing off the coffee table or doing a few minutes of gentle stretching. Remember that your day is not all or nothing—a tidied coffee table makes for a tidier home, even if the dishes are piled up in the sink. Focusing on these small accomplishments can help you feel less frazzled and out of control.

Sometimes the most direct route to a feeling of mastery is to do something that you're really good at. (This is a kind of self-care, right up there with showering and seeing your friends.) One of our patients, a cellist, told us, "I didn't play at all at the end of my pregnancy (I could barely reach the bow around my belly) and wasn't sure if I should go back to my community orchestra after the baby was born. I couldn't make it to a lot of rehearsals, and made a lot of mistakes, but once I got back into it, I realized that I had been doing this my whole life before becoming a mom. Playing music gives me a rush and sense of accomplishment that I never get after a day of taking care of the baby, so it felt really good to remember how that feels."

Every day, your list of priorities may change. Some days, the only thing on your list for the day will be to SURVIVE. As one of our patients said, "Learn how to tolerate that you can't do it all. If you finish a day and think, *What have I accomplished?* remember you've accomplished a lot if you kept your baby alive, fed, and clean-ish."

Clean-*ish*, not clean. Experienced mothers will tell you: You're going to have to get comfortable with things being messy. And when we say messy, we're talking figuratively and literally. Babies go through diapers, wipes, clothes, and sometimes bedding at a dizzying rate. If you're bottle-feeding, then bottles, nipples, pump parts, and formula will take over your cupboards and counter space. No matter how big your house is or how much of a minimalist you are, it may seem like a baby's "stuff" takes over before she's even old enough to play with toys. Unless you have household help *and* help with the baby (and sometimes even when you do), you may need to let your standards for clutter and cleanliness slide a little.

This can be especially difficult for those of us who feel comforted and calmed by a well-managed home, especially when the rest of life feels out of control. Focus on small changes you can make, and remember that a little cleaning is better than none. And when you say to yourself, *It's four p.m., I* should *have cleaned the house already today*, where is that coming from? Often, you're comparing yourself to an idealized image of another mother's life. Trust us, most new mothers imagine that others are "doing it better." When you see another mother on the street and feel subpar, remind yourself that some chaos in early motherhood is universal, even if you can't see it from the outside.

Tackling "Should Statements"

In cognitive behavioral therapy (CBT), we encourage patients to look at patterns in the language they use when they narrate their own thoughts throughout the day. The word "should" is a red flag that you may be putting unhealthy pressure on yourself, thinking in terms of self-criticism. "Should statements" tend to demoralize rather than motivate and inspire.

CBT research shows that monitoring and rephrasing your "should statements" can help reduce feelings of shame and keep a distorted perspective in check. The following exercise may be helpful: Every time you say or think "should" about a parenting task, write down that statement. After you write down your "should statement," on the line below, write down a new, positive, generous thought. Perhaps you can think of how you might respond to a friend if she shared her negative "should statement." It may help to jot these thoughts down in the moment when you catch yourself thinking them, then to sit down later, when you have some free time, and rephrase them in a more self-loving light.

Here are some examples:

1. **Should statement:** "The baby finally fell asleep. I want to crawl into bed without even brushing my teeth, but I **should** go finish the dishes."

   Positive reframe: "It took forever to get the baby to sleep. I'm exhausted and need to recover for the next round when she wakes up. My daughter needs me to be well rested so I can be more present with her, but she doesn't even know what dishes are, let alone that the dirty ones are sitting in the sink. I'm the only one who will probably notice that there are dishes in the sink, so maybe I can live with that and get some rest."

2. **Should statement:** "My friends are coming over to meet the baby. I **should** get some snacks and drinks out for them—they're always such great hosts when I visit them."

   Positive reframe: "My friends are coming over, and they know I'm still recovering from my C-section and am alone with the baby. I can suggest they bring some snacks with them—they know that in general, I'm a generous host, but today I'm not myself."

3. **Should statement:** "I **should** make my bed every morning—it's so lazy not to."

   Positive reframe: "I'll try making my bed to see if it helps me feel happier and more organized. But time when the baby naps is limited, and it's more important for me to take a shower. I'm not lazy, I'm just really busy and need to prioritize what's most important."

Sharing the Care: The Early Postpartum and Your Partner

If you're partnered, your family has now grown from two to three. While the transition feels different for each couple (and each partner), we can pretty much guarantee that having a baby will change your relationship. Until now, you may have shared significant milestones like a wedding, responsibilities like the care of a dog, and routines like the management of your home. But you've never shared an experience like parenting. Now that you're parenting together, you are family in a new way.

You may find the experience to be bonding for you and your partner as you encounter challenges, intensities, and responsibilities together. But as with any big change in a relationship, it will take some effort to figure out your new normal. As a couple, you will have to renegotiate your roles and routines to include the baby, both physically and psychologically, within your home and your lives.

We hope your partner will be with you full-time for a few weeks after the baby is born. Lean on her—literally. If you need help getting up and going to the bathroom or up the stairs, or you need her to hold the baby so you can get some sleep after a two a.m. feeding, ask. You may feel embarrassed or upset that you have to be so dependent. Remember that you're a team—you'll be there for her when she's vulnerable, too.

One of our patients gave this helpful advice: "It wasn't really so different from other times in our marriage—we sort of have this rule that only one of us is allowed to fall apart at a time; the other has to keep it together, and then they can let go later. In the first few weeks after I had the baby, it was clear I was going to be the one who was a mess, but we both knew that eventually, I'd be there once again as his rock. It's always a give-and-take."

You may be pleasantly surprised by how intuitive, nurturing, and adaptable your partner is; you may enjoy getting to know a different side of him as a father (or her as a mother). One of our patients shared how having a baby brought out her husband's "maternal" side: "I was recovering from a birth injury and had a hard time walking around the house and picking up the baby. I was anxious about how to take care of the baby and was still in pain. My husband really stepped up and was the first one to jump up when the baby was crying. He kept track of the feeding and pooping and sleeping in the first few weeks, because I could barely manage those things for myself."

Sometimes, even when your needs—or the baby's needs—are obvious to you, your partner may not see what you see, so it will be important to ask for help directly. **Don't expect your partner to be a mind reader.** While it would be lovely to have your needs taken care of before you ask, it's better to ask than to resent your partner's lack of psychic ability. We recommend that you try to be as specific and as practical as you can about what you need, even if you think it's obvious. If you want him to buy diapers, don't assume he knows what brand or what size.

One of our patients told us, "I usually did the laundry, but when I was busy with the baby, I realized I couldn't keep up with my usual share of the chores. For a while I thought my husband would notice and offer to do it—I certainly would have—but he was oblivious to the dirty clothes piling up in the hamper. At first I was annoyed. I was keeping track of everything that the baby needed, why wasn't it obvious to him that he should take care of our meals and lives so that I could take care of her? Rather than staying mad I decided to be direct and just said, 'You need to take over doing the laundry.' He didn't miss a beat and just started doing it. I'm glad I didn't pick a fight."

Another one of our patients had a harder time keeping her cool, especially when she was exhausted: "As a couple, we've always been great communicators, but the first four weeks were really hard. My husband felt like I was being overbearing when I ran to pick up our daughter at her first cry, and I thought he was being insensitive when he didn't jump up right away. I felt guilty because he's so supportive and giving, but sometimes I just blew up and said, 'You're doing it all wrong!' I know it hurt his feelings."

New Parenting and Your Relationship: Communication Skills 101

The best thing you can do for your relationship during this demanding transition is to communicate, with sensitivity, about what you're feeling and what you need from each other. This was true even before you had a baby, but it's always hard to do, because it requires you to share your vulnerable feelings and be interested in your partner's, even if you don't understand them. These tips may be new to you, or just a reminder to be mindful of them in this challenging time:

- **Don't respond in the heat of the moment.** If you're frustrated with your partner, wait to talk until your initial anger has passed. Expressing the fact that you're angry is less important than talking about what made you angry and working together to keep it from happening again. If you're in transit, both tired and hungry, or navigating some challenge with the baby, write down what you want to say and then find a better time to say it than when you're both overwhelmed.

- **Just listening is often enough.** If your partner is a problem-solver, you might start by saying, "I just want you to listen."

Explain that talking is a good way for you to vent, and that a complaint doesn't mean you're implying it's your partner's fault or that he needs to fix it. If your partner is coming to you with a problem, try to listen with genuine curiosity and ask how you can be more supportive, rather than using the opportunity to defend yourself. Remember that the goal isn't being right, it's being a better team.

- **Talk about your roles.** Ideally, before having children, you set aside time to talk about the caretaking roles you would each like to assume in the family, but it's always good to continue (or begin) the conversation. Important topics are: gender roles, financial choices, career paths, disciplinary style, and who will handle meals, mornings, and bedtime. Whether child care is evenly shared or one parent takes on more of the work, the division of responsibility should be agreed to consciously and collaboratively.

- **Share stories about your own childhood.** Telling each other how you were raised, down to the nitty-gritty, will help you better understand your partner and may clarify disagreements. You may be surprised by your differences of perspective and learn new things about your partner's history of warm memories and wounds.

- **Unpack any resentment that precedes parenting.** One of our patients was the primary breadwinner in her family. Before having a baby, she felt burdened by this financial pressure, and when she became a mother, the feelings only intensified. It's important to find a calm way to talk about these resentments and how you'd like to adjust your roles.

- **Speak from the "I."** You may be familiar with "I feel" statements as a communication tool. It's not just about starting with "I feel," though. If you said, "I feel frustrated when you change her diaper because you do it wrong," that would still be accusatory and trigger your partner's defensiveness. Really speaking from the "I" includes naming your feelings *and* taking responsibility for them.

- **Be constructive with your criticism.** There's a difference between "Would you please do more diaper changes?" and "Why do you never do anything for the baby?" Instead of focusing on your partner's shortcomings, look toward the future and ask for the specific changes she needs in order to succeed at helping you.

- **Talk to your partner as if she's a stranger.** We often make the mistake of believing that if we love someone, then we don't have to rely on the same kind of politeness we use to communicate in the workplace or with acquaintances. It may seem counter-intuitive in a relationship that demands emotional honesty to thrive, but social niceties help to prevent defensiveness and hurt feelings. Remembering to say "please" and "thank you" goes a long way.

Supportive Co-parenting

There's an old saying that in a good marriage, you're each giving 60 percent. If you are partnered, there are many times in the life of a relationship, especially parenting, when you may feel like the responsibilities aren't being evenly divided. Maybe one of you feels more pressure with child care, while the other feels more financial pressure. Add centuries of cultural ideas about gender roles and parenting, and it's not so obvious how to share the load.

These days, fathers may be more involved in child care than in generations past. However, even in dual-earning families, studies show that mothers are often still viewed as "the natural parenting experts," leaving fathers to take on a helpful but secondary role. A 2015 Pew Research Center survey shows that in two-parent families, parenting and household responsibilities are shared more equally when both the mother and father work full-time, but a larger share of the day-to-day parenting responsibilities often falls to mothers. This phenomenon has been studied in both married and unmarried relationships, and parenting imbalances crop up in same-sex couples, too.

Supportive co-parenting is a concept that can be helpful for parents thinking about how to balance the emotional and practical labor at home. The term was first used to help with parenting after divorce, but now it's being used to help all couples better work together as a team. Supportive co-parenting is defined as when both parents share overlapping practical and emotional responsibilities for caretaking of children, openly communicate about their strategies and feelings in these roles, and support each other's efforts. **Supportive co-parenting isn't about splitting the work of child care down the middle; instead its about feeling emotionally supported by your partner in the shared experience of parenting.** Another key aspect of supportive co-parenting is an openness to reevaluate the balance of your domestic roles over time. Translation: Discussions about changing the diapers, taking out the garbage, and rocking a colicky baby will be part of your calm and weekly conversations, not whispered in resentful digs or screamed during brawls.

Studies show what you can probably guess: The long-term practice of supportive co-parenting can have positive psychological benefits for each of you, your relationship, and your children. It can improve the quality of your parenting and enhance your relationship satisfaction and marital health, even decreasing your frequency of fighting and risk of divorce.

As much as you may want more help from your partner, it can sometimes be difficult to share the decision-making. As one of our patients described: "I hated it when he would come home from work and give me advice on how to get the baby to sleep. I wanted to say, 'I've been at this all day. You should be asking me what to do, not telling me you know better.'" You may resent your partner walking into the situation and asserting control over your "territory." But your partner may feel like he has something valuable to contribute and doesn't want to be relegated to a supporting role or dismissed as a know-nothing.

If you've carried the pregnancy, and if you're now breastfeeding, you and your baby have been physically connected—your partner hasn't been a part of that. He may feel left out of or excluded from the parenting experience. Now that the baby is here, your partner may have been expecting to get some of you back—emotionally and physically—but instead, all your attention is going to the baby. Your partner may have a hard time being supportive and involved in co-parenting if his feelings are hurt. He may not even realize that he's feeling neglected (and sleep- and sex-deprived), but you may see it in his irritability or feel it in his distance.

Reconnecting in Your Relationship

One of our patients told us about the first time she realized how hard it was to be mindful of her relationship when she was exhausted from taking care of the baby: "One night when my baby was a few weeks old, my husband came home from work and wanted to tell me about his day, but it was hard to focus while I was feeding the baby. After I finally got the baby to sleep, I was so excited to sit on the couch and watch TV, just zone out and have my first real break of the day. But as soon as we sat down, my husband put his arm around me and started rubbing my arm. I flinched away. I didn't even know why, I just couldn't handle being touched. He got angry because he thought I was being rude, which I thought was unfair, though I guess I understand that he just wanted us to be close and have some adult time, to cuddle or just sit together and talk, but I couldn't handle it after spending all day with the baby attached to me."

We hear stories like this from new mothers all the time. It's common to find your desire to be alone confusing, especially when you normally find comfort in being close to your partner. But if you're at the end of an exhausting stretch of holding the baby all day, you may want some physical space for yourself. It's not about pushing your partner away but about simply needing to take care of yourself before you can feel human again, let alone sexy. It's important that you communicate this to your partner so that you can be mindful of her feelings around intimacy and rejection.

Often in relationships, people pick fights because, even unconsciously, they feel invisible and abandoned. Knowing that your intimate time as a couple isn't over, just postponed for the moment, can help you both be more patient with everyday struggles.

Taking stock of how your relationship routine has changed will help you keep an eye out for when you can return to the rituals and routines that make you "feel like you" as a couple. **As with your own self-care, make a list of your relationship self-care items to keep as a reminder.** If you normally talk about the day over dinner, be mindful of the baby's sleep schedule so that you can have at least one meal a day together—maybe it's breakfast instead of dinner. Plan date ideas that you can look forward to a few weeks down the road. Ask a family member or babysitter to watch the kids so you can go out for the type of date you used to enjoy before parenthood. Make plans with other adults to reconnect as a couple in a social setting.

It may also help to encourage your partner to maintain his

relationships with other adults so that he has a wide circle of support, rather than leaning on only your marriage for his social, emotional, and recreational needs. This, of course, requires making yourself available to watch the baby so that he can go out—but he should be doing the same for you. Swap off on child care so that you encourage each other to exercise, socialize, and take care of yourselves. The more outlets you each have, the more bandwidth you'll have to support each other and your baby.

Visitors

As soon as you tell people you've had your baby, they may start asking to come visit. It's only natural—they want to meet your new family member and shower you with love. You need community and your extended support system, too, but it's important to be deliberate about how and when you welcome visitors.

Hosting guests when you've just had a baby—and for as long as it takes for you to feel back to normal—is not like having guests over at other times. **Your job is to take care of your baby and to let your partner and visitors take care of you.** This means not worrying about the state of your living room, whether you've put on mascara, or whether your sister's favorite soda is in the fridge. If guests ask, "What can I bring?" answer honestly—maybe it would be helpful for them to bring food or the dishwasher detergent you haven't had a chance to buy. Welcoming guests to your home is usually a generous act, but now is the time to be a little bit selfish.

A friend told us, "However many visitors you were thinking you wanted to have in a day, take that number down one. The act of even talking to other people is exhausting in the beginning. It's okay to ask someone to leave in five minutes or tell people you don't want them to come over for a while. If you struggle with this, ask your partner to play bad cop by asking your guests to leave. Or give your friends advance warning in a text, like: 'I tend to get tired after fifteen minutes, so that may be all I can handle, but I still want you to come if you're up for a short visit.'"

Also be prepared for a shift in dynamic from your pregnancy. Your friends may have been very tuned in to your needs and comfort during the pregnancy, but now that the baby is here, you may no longer be the main attraction. You may feel proud but neglected. You can use this to your advantage—if your friend is obsessed with your fussy baby, and you're comfortable doing so, let her rock him while you grab a quick shower. She'll get the experience of bonding with the baby while you take advantage of the extra hands.

You can't predict which of your friends will or won't want to visit in these early weeks. A friend who miscarried may avoid coming over to visit because seeing your baby would be painful for her. Another who always proclaimed her dislike of children may be first in line to visit, bringing snacks and gifts and helping you fold laundry. The best thing you can do is set aside expectations and let your friends take the lead. Eventually, you'll want to make sure the relationships that matter to you stay intact, but in the first several weeks, you should be focusing more on your own needs than theirs.

If you have very demanding friends, you may want to politely postpone having them over until you've recovered your energy and are more comfortable with your baby. The only people you should welcome into your home at this time are those who won't burden you with their issues or prioritize their emotions over yours. One of our patients said, "My friends brought their son, who had a cough. I pulled my husband into the nursery and told him I was worried about our baby getting sick. We came back into the living room, and I realized that they had heard us on the monitor. At first I was mortified, but then I realized I was relieved that they heard me and left. It was what I wanted all along. Why was I so afraid of asking for it directly in my own home?"

Visitors Checklist

Who comes and how long they stay is up to you and your partner. It's your baby and your boundaries. Decide together ahead of time:

- How many visitors are you comfortable with per day?
- Are some people welcome and others not?
- Are we setting a time limit on visits?
- Who is allowed to hold the baby?
- Are we comfortable with the baby being photographed? Or us? Can they post the images on social media?
- If you're nursing, will you breastfeed in front of other people?
- If someone has a cold, can she visit?
- Do you want everyone to wash their hands before holding the baby? Or leave their shoes at the door? Who will enforce that rule?

If your family lives close to you, you may find yourself spending more time than usual around your mother and/or stepmom and/or mother-in-law. Even if you don't live close to each other, don't be surprised if your family travels to see you and the newest member of the family more frequently. If you had clearly drawn boundaries with your families before, the arrival of a baby can break those down.

As one of our patients shared: "Some grandparents think they own the baby, so you do have to be a little careful. You're still in charge. Authority gets confusing." Another told this story: "My father-in-law kept trying to teach my newborn daughter to call him 'Duke' because he hates the word 'grandpa.' It makes me so angry—my daughter wasn't even talking yet, and this is his focus when he comes over? Even with a new child in the family, my father-in-law continues to think he's the center of the universe."

Just because they are now grandparents, your or your partner's parents probably won't magically transform into different versions of themselves. If your mom was never terribly nurturing, she may be less into cuddling your baby and more focused on vacuuming the house. If your mother-in-law tends to ignore you and fawn over your partner, giving her a grandchild probably won't change anything.

On the other hand, you may be pleasantly surprised. Maybe your partner's mother, who has always been cool and critical of you, is supportive of your choice to bottle-feed. As one of our patients shared: "I became a lot closer with my mother-in-law after my daughter was born. I think it was really helpful for us to have something in common. We're from different countries and cultures, so it had been really hard for us to find a point of connection before the baby."

Sometimes grandparents grow into their new roles gradually; sometimes they reject them or see them differently than you do. You're allowed to be hurt and disappointed, even if it has nothing to do with the baby. As one of our patients described: "My parents were so loving with the baby—they were just obsessed with her. It was so different from how I remembered my childhood—they were so overwhelmed by my brother, who was sick, that I don't remember them doting on me like that. It made me sad to realize that they were better grandparents then they were parents to me." If you feel up to it, consider sharing your observations with your parents. You can start by complimenting them on how warm and emotionally available they are as grandparents, by way of opening up a dialogue about how their experience as grandparents compares to their own experience as parents. If it feels right to share any painful memories or questions from your childhood with them, consider it. They may have enough distance now to offer an apology or an explanation.

Family members will often visit and bring with them the (unwelcome) gift of unsolicited advice. While these tips from an older sister, cousin, mother, or mother-in-law are usually backed by good intentions, there can be an undertone of "I know better than you; I'm the real mom in this family." You may feel that members of your family are being condescending because of your inexperience and not taking your maternal authority seriously. Part of your psychological task of creating a new identity in your matrescence is to give yourself time to trust your own decisions and accept your maternal authority. Even if the advice makes sense, if it doesn't fit your parenting style, then it's not right for you.

If you're trying to avoid a potentially inflammatory confrontation with a family matriarch, you can try saying, "Thanks for the advice," or, "That's a great story." You certainly don't have to do what they recommend, or announce that you won't.

If these conversations involve your partner's family—or if they don't—knowing your partner will back you up, or join you in giving the message, is important. If you're feeling like your husband is deferring to his parents' comfort before yours, try to find the time to talk to him in private about how this is making you feel.

One of our patients said, "My husband's parents are so controlling—every time we see them, it has to be in their house, on their terms, with their schedule. I usually just deal with it, and he seems to see it from their side, saying, 'They're just trying to make a nice dinner for us; they prepared all day,' if I ever complain. But I can't keep disrupting the baby's schedule and driving out there when I know there will be traffic on the way home and I have to work the next morning. I had to explain to him that we needed to sometimes say no to them to keep the baby in her routine—even if it meant disappointing them."

Remember that your partner's dynamic with his parents is probably a long-standing survival strategy for him. Just like you, he has had to negotiate his emotions and emotional disappointments with his parents his whole life. He may be tolerant or dismissive of their bad behavior because he has learned how to focus on the good and ignore the bad with them for years. So rather than trying to convince him to change the way he sees them, it's usually more constructive to focus on what you need and why it's best for your whole family, especially the baby.

Caring for Your Newborn—and Yourself

Feeding

Whether it's with breast milk, formula, or a combination of both, every mother and baby will need to figure out the feeding choices that work best for them.

In the hours and first few days after childbirth, you may have received breastfeeding advice from a nurse, doula, or lactation consultant. Most women find that breastfeeding involves a learning curve, though some find it comes easily. It can take days or weeks for you and your baby to navigate your way.

Since some cultures send such a strong message about the health benefits of breastfeeding, many moms feel proud when breastfeeding is going well—like they have passed their first important test of motherhood with flying colors. The emotional experience of being able to give your baby exactly what she needs—food and cuddling—can be tremendously gratifying. Babies are hard to figure out and often difficult to soothe, but when they're hungry and want to be fed, they can become relaxed and fully content within moments. Being able to make that happen with your own body can feel like an exhilarating superpower, especially as your baby matures and becomes more challenging to soothe in other ways. That being said, not every woman can or wants to breastfeed. While the benefits of breastfeeding are seen in scientific literature, in our clinical experience, our patients tell us that the differences for their babies (even mothers who have given one baby formula and the other breast milk) may be imperceptible. **Breastfeeding is not nature's way of testing your abilities as a mother, and formula feeding is not any indication of failure or insufficiency.**

Many women admit to us that, even when it works, breastfeeding can sometimes be hard. It can be painful for your nipples and difficult for the baby to latch. This can become frustrating and exhausting, especially in the middle of the night, when you're the only one who can do the feeds because you're the only one with the boobs. And sometimes, no matter how hard you try, it just doesn't work. If your goal is to breastfeed, we recommend asking your provider for help or seeking out a lactation consultant or breastfeeding support group (see **Resources**). Sometimes your pediatrician can advise how to help the baby with latch or other issues. We know many moms who were ultimately able to enjoy breastfeeding after getting past the initial hump.

If you're struggling with breastfeeding, your doctor may advise you to try giving your baby a bottle of pumped breast milk or supplementing with formula. Sometimes—for example, if you have a low supply—supplementing with formula for a period of time may actually help with breastfeeding. Otherwise, your baby may not get enough food, and she may become increasingly agitated or too tired to work on breastfeeding. You may become burned out from the pressure, too. If you supplement with formula, you may be able to take your time and ultimately have more patience to give breastfeeding a shot.

We think that the social pressure on new mothers to breastfeed can be psychologically burdensome at times. If you experience more stress than satisfaction from breastfeeding, it makes sense to explore your alternatives. If breastfeeding isn't working well for you or your baby, you may choose to exclusively pump so that you can still provide breast milk to your baby. Or, you may decide to supplement with or switch fully to formula. (Of course, bottle-feeding is not without its challenges. You may have to try several nipples before you find one that your baby likes. Formula, too, is not one-size-fits-all; you may have to try several different kinds before you find the one that works best for your baby's digestion.)

The wellness of your baby depends on several factors including: feeding, sleeping, and bonding. If using formula helps your baby get more calories and sleep for longer stretches, that's a good thing. And if formula helps you to be calmer and more emotionally present during feeds and overall, then it may very well be more beneficial for your child's health by facilitating your attachment.

Breastfeeding also continues the connection between your body to your baby's. While some women find this to be a pleasurable assistance in bonding, for others, it feels like a constraint. If you're sensitive to the feeling that pregnancy made your body stop being yours, and that the disparity of demands on you as compared to your partner were unfair, a long period of breastfeeding may not make sense for you. Many of the women we speak with enjoy breastfeeding for a few months, but then ask for our "permission" to stop before a year because they feel guilty about switching to formula. Other women we speak with enjoy breastfeeding beyond twelve months and experience an inverse pressure from family, friends, or even doctors who may ask, "Why haven't you stopped yet?"

Food is often an emotionally charged topic in families, and how you feed your baby is not an exception. Your mother may have breastfed you, and she may be judgmental of your decision to switch to formula for night feeds so you can sleep. Or you may be struggling to breastfeed and feel hurt by your mother's callous disregard of your efforts when she says she never breastfed you and what's the big deal. You can choose to keep your feeding decisions private, and you don't need to take anyone's input. On the other hand, you may find that openness leads the way to surprisingly helpful conversations. One patient told us, "I was struggling with breastfeeding, and I felt like such a failure. My mom always pushed me to be an overachiever, so I was worried about telling her. But when I did, she was so understanding. She told me that she hadn't been able to breastfeed me at all. I was relieved that she wasn't judgmental, and it also reminded me that people—like me—turn out totally fine on formula, too."

Whether you choose to breastfeed or bottle-feed, there will probably come a time when you have to feed in public. In the United States, nursing mothers are protected by law and allowed to breastfeed in public. We encourage you to feed any way that makes you feel the most comfortable, whatever that means to you. And you may need to reevaluate in different situations. For example, you may be comfortable breastfeeding in front of a stranger, but not your father (or vice versa). However, some people may view feeding your child out in the open as inappropriate—you may receive stares, disapproving looks, or even unwelcome comments. And if you're bottle-feeding, strangers may share their opinions or unsolicited advice. As with reactions to your pregnant body from strangers, it's up to you how you respond. We encourage you to do what feels best for you, ranging from ignoring them, to smiling and nodding, to rolling your eyes, to giving them an unsolicited lecture about unsolicited advice.

The best advice *we* can give you is to remind yourself that no matter what happens, your baby will grow out of this phase, and you'll have a lifetime of being able to feed your child in other ways. One of our patients who was unable to breastfeed felt disappointed that feeding her baby with formula was "unnatural." When her baby was old enough to start solids, she approached making homemade organic baby food with gusto, which improved her self-esteem about being a "natural" nurturer. While some moms would find it a burden to shop, prepare, and purée food that could alternately be picked up at the grocery store, this mother found the process of food preparation to be therapeutic.

Sleep

Before you became a mother, you probably pulled all-nighters, pushed through jet lag, or tossed and turned because you were upset or kept awake by noisy neighbors. But no matter how grueling the circumstances, you were probably able to get a good night's sleep at some point. When you have a new baby, it's like *Groundhog Day* for sleep deprivation—for the first few weeks, even months, a good night's sleep may never come.

Every adult requires a different amount of sleep, but each of us has a point when we will start to feel sick, physically and emotionally, if we aren't getting enough. Sleep deprivation makes it hard to think straight and can interfere with your memory, concentration, and ability to make good decisions. It can lower your energy (not to mention sex drive), raise your blood pressure, cause mood swings and irritability, and wreak havoc on your body by increasing your stress hormones. We've worked with patients whose sleep deprivation has contributed to postpartum depression and some who told us that it interfered with their breast milk supply as well.

Adrenaline, caffeine, and love for your new baby may keep you going in the short term, but they cannot replace high-quality sleep. In fact, when new moms come to our offices for help, the very first question we ask about is their sleep. We've even been known to write "SLEEP" on a prescription pad and send our patients home with strict instructions. We don't recommend this because it's an easy fix. **It's just that time and time again, we've seen that problems with mood and anxiety can improve with a few good nights of sleep.** When sleep is not restored, postpartum depression or other psychological challenges are more likely to follow.

Expert opinions differ on this, but we advise our patients to aim for at least one block of four consecutive hours of sleep at night. Naps help, but they don't make up completely for lack of quality sleep at night. The popular advice to "nap when the baby naps" is logical, but turning off your mind to sleep just because your body is fatigued and the baby is down is much easier said than done. Anyone who has ever had insomnia will be able to understand how that feeling of time pressure makes it hard to relax. And failing to time your naps to the baby's can be another trigger for feeling like a failure.

In our experience, the best relief will come from asking for help with at least one nighttime feed from your partner, a family member, a friend, or a child care professional so that she can feed the baby a pumped or formula bottle while you get a few extra hours of sleep. Or, if you're exclusively nursing, she can bring you the baby for feeding and take over changing diapers and other care.

If you or your partner is a night owl or an early bird, you can divide the night's child care in half and let the other sleep four hours in a row. Maybe you could take the late-night session, and your partner could crash early and get up for the five a.m. "wake-up call" or vice versa.

Feedings are one impediment to good sleep, but even when your baby is fast asleep in her crib in the middle of the night, you may find yourself unable to relax. Just knowing about the possibility of sudden infant death syndrome (SIDS) is a source of universal anxiety for parents. It is one of the reasons many parents are hypervigilant and more anxious at night. The risk of SIDS is greatest in the first six months of life, and while SIDS is very rare, the fear can persist and be a common source of nighttime stress for parents.

The current APA recommendations (see **Resources**) suggest that the baby should sleep in your room, but in his own safely arranged bassinette or crib, for the first six months to a year. Some mothers find having the baby next to them at night to be reassuring. If you're nursing, it may be easier for everyone to get back to sleep after the night feeds when you're all in the same room.

Other mothers, however, find it difficult to sleep well with the baby in their room. Evolution may explain why so many new mothers are highly sensitive to their babies' movements and noises. There are benefits to being primed to be so alert, but if you're woken up by every tiny sound, and you find yourself lying awake listening to your baby's breath, this may not work well in the long term. If sleeping next to the baby makes you too keyed up to sleep (and you have space) think about sleeping in another room away from the baby during your "hours off," and maybe using earplugs so that you can get some uninterrupted rest while your partner is on duty. (Same goes for a baby monitor—if you find yourself lying awake staring at it when you could and should otherwise be sleeping, talk to your pediatrician about what's best for your whole family's health.)

However you arrange your and your baby's night routine, we hope you will remember that flexibility and adaptability are important. As with all other aspects of child care, it's good to reassess your decisions when you feel like they are causing more stress than benefit. Changing your mind is not a sign of weakness; think of it as an indication that you're learning from experience and adapting to your baby's evolving needs. If you need or want to experiment with your sleeping arrangements, talk to your pediatrician and, with her approval, do it. Things will probably change again in a few weeks— or days or months—as your baby grows, her brain matures, and her sleep patterns change.

Leaving the Nest

Staying home and cocooning with your baby, especially in the first week or two, can be restorative. It gives you the chance to physically recover, practice feeding or nursing, develop confidence in your mastery of the new skills of child care, and let your baby adjust to life outside the womb without being overstimulated. As long as you're not feeling isolated and lonely, it can be cozy and beneficial.

But at some point, you will have to leave the house. It's not physically, psychologically, or socially healthy for you to be quarantined at home for too long without vitamin D from sunlight and stimulation from the sights, sounds, and interactions of the adult world. Besides, you and your baby will have to get to doctors' appointments and become mobile so that you can maintain some self-sufficiency and not have to completely depend on others to bring the outside world to you.

If you're hesitant about leaving home with the baby, try to figure out why you're reluctant. Do you simply need a little more time to recover your strength, or are you physically ready but emotionally hesitant? Are you anxious about forgetting some of your baby care supplies? Are you afraid something will happen to the baby? That he'll start crying and you won't be able to calm him? Figuring out what's underneath your sense of anxiety or resistance is important.

Fear is often at the root of these new experiences. One of our patients told us, "I felt a pit in my stomach the first time I crossed the street with my baby. I realized that it was the first time out in the world that she was outside my body *and* outside my protection. A bike could hit her, the stroller wheel could break. It's so scary, because as much as you try, you can't control the world that your baby is in now." When this patient was at home, she had anticipatory anxiety, meaning that when she imagined leaving the house, all she could think about were worst-case scenarios. This patient was very anxious about going outside alone with her baby, but after a few times, she saw that nothing bad happened, and her catastrophic worries started to fade.

If you're worried about your baby getting upset in public, try to give yourself permission to be a beginner, and know that it's okay to fumble and learn in public. Everyone knows that babies cry, and when yours does, you're not ruining anyone's day or branding yourself as a terrible mother. As one of our patients came to understand: **"Out in the world, no one is thinking about you or judging you as much as you are thinking about and judging yourself.** Strangers on the street know how to ignore a crying baby." And if someone *is* thinking critical thoughts about you—what's actually the harm? It's in his head; it doesn't have to be in yours.

Start small. Your baby's first few weeks probably aren't the best time for an eight-hour train ride to see Grandma. If all you feel up to is a walk to the end of the block or a half hour in the backyard, that's fine. Next time, go a little farther. Take the baby on short errands or for a walk in the park. It may not be realistic to try to coordinate your trip with the baby's feeding times or naps early on; he's still too unpredictable. Take your time getting ready. Make sure you have everything you think you'll need while you're gone, but remind yourself that if you forget something, you can always wing it or turn around and come home. If you feel more secure with a companion, enlist your partner or a friend to go with you. Do your best to prepare for the unexpected, and be willing to change your plans if you're uncomfortable being around someone with a cold, a diaper overflows, or your baby has a meltdown. The more times you go out, and the farther afield you go, the more confidence you'll feel.

Just as it's important to leave the house with your baby, it's important to venture out without her, too. One of our patients admitted how good it felt to go off on her own, truly solo for the first time, in, well, about three months: "I left my husband with formula and all the other supplies and went to the dentist, and to buy a new bra. I felt bad, but I didn't miss the baby at all. It felt awesome to have some time to myself, get some fresh air, and get something accomplished." When she came back home, she felt refreshed and happier to be with her baby after enjoying herself on her humble solo adventure.

Leaving your baby for the first time can be nerve-racking—you've basically never been apart before. Think of ways to make yourself feel more at ease. Maybe you would feel better if your partner, or mother, or partner *and* mother were there in your absence. Maybe the only person you trust right now is your best friend, who's a mother of three. Or, if you have hired a babysitter or baby nurse, you may be reassured by knowing that she is a child care professional trained in CPR. Once you get over the hump of these early separations, you will learn to be more trusting of a responsible person.

Also know that you don't have to enjoy your first few experiences apart from your baby. It's natural to feel emotional about early separations. As one of our patients described: "I remember the first time my husband and I left the house to go out to dinner. I felt so much pressure, like *I'm supposed to be having fun*. But I was so tired I could barely get through the meal. I trusted my parents to care for the baby but couldn't enjoy myself because I kept thinking, *What's the baby doing? Does he need me?* The next time she and her husband went out to dinner, she was much more relaxed. It may take a couple of outings until you're able to enjoy yourself, too.

You and your partner may have different opinions and priorities about separations from the baby. It's one of those issues that may bring up feelings rooted in your past childhood experiences and therefore may require some thoughtful communication and reflection. These disagreements can become the flashpoint for an argument if you don't take the time to explain where you're coming from. One of our patients told us, "I was basically raised by my older stepsister because my parents were never home. I never want my child to feel that I care more about being with others than I do about her. I needed to explain to my wife that it wasn't that I didn't care about our date night, I just knew I would have more fun if I put the baby down myself before we went out. She was disappointed to be heading out so late, but I promised her I would bring my portable pump so that we could stay out as late as we wanted and have a good time together."

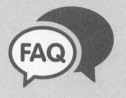 Everyone's first few months of parenthood are different. Here are a few of the most common questions we hear:

Aside from routine appointments, when should you call the pediatrician?

In terms of straight-up health issues or medical questions, your first call should be to your pediatrician. If you're worried about a rash, a fever, or your baby's reaction to a medication, call the doctor. She will be able to tell you if you should bring your baby in or wait things out.

Even if you're worried that she won't take you seriously if you're calling frequently just to calm your own anxiety, call her. You may in fact need to work on why you're so anxious, but that's a separate issue. It's her and her staff's job to deal with anxious parents; you won't be the first. It's not your job to suffer silently and worry that there's something seriously wrong with your child.

Several of our patients have talked to us about conflict they felt with their pediatricians. One woman said, "I met with a pediatrician when I was pregnant who spent the whole time talking about breastfeeding and how it's the best thing you can do for your baby. I wasn't sure I wanted to breastfeed and wanted a pediatrician who was a better listener rather than rushing in and out and blurting instructions. I realized this doctor was just too intense for me."

If your pediatrician and her staff make you feel bad for calling and being concerned, then you may want to find a different doctor.

As with an obstetric practitioner, there are many different styles of pediatricians. **Your gut is as important as a doctor's online rating.** You should trust his expertise and how he approaches the patient-doctor relationship, and feel that his child care philosophies are consistent with your approach.

How do I help my older child adjust when I bring the new baby home?

It's normal for an older sibling to feel jealous of the new baby. But even if your older child isn't expressing jealousy, you may find that her behavior regresses. A toddler who was toilet trained may wet the bed or demand a bottle of her own. If she recently switched to a big-kid bed, she may want to get back into her old crib. An older child may act out because he wants attention of any kind, good or bad.

One way to make your older child feel included is to give him a baby doll or stuffed animal. You can encourage and praise his parallel play with his baby doll: "You're feeding your baby so nicely!" Applaud your child for being a great big brother, and for how gentle he is around the baby. You can involve your older child in caring for the baby by asking him to hand you a diaper, or keep you company and snuggle while you feed the baby. Point out things your older child can do that the baby can't, and applaud him for it. Also, encourage special big-kid activities with your partner while you're home with the baby or vice versa. If you're not partnered, grandparents, friends, or a child care professional can take the same role.

When you praise or include your older child in the baby's care,

you're helping to foster a positive sibling relationship. In part, this is because you're continuing to give your older child plenty of positive attention. It's normal for her to feel displaced or jealous of the attention the baby is receiving. If she can't articulate her upset feelings in words, she may act them out by being mean or rough with her teddy bear. Don't be alarmed; expressing her feelings in "play" can be a healthy way for her to deal with frustration. You can't take away her negative feelings, nor should you.

If you see this happening, you can help by asking questions, such as, "Are you mad that I have to take care of the baby?" Let your older child know that it's okay to feel angry—and okay to be rough with her dolls as make-believe—but not okay to be rough with the baby.

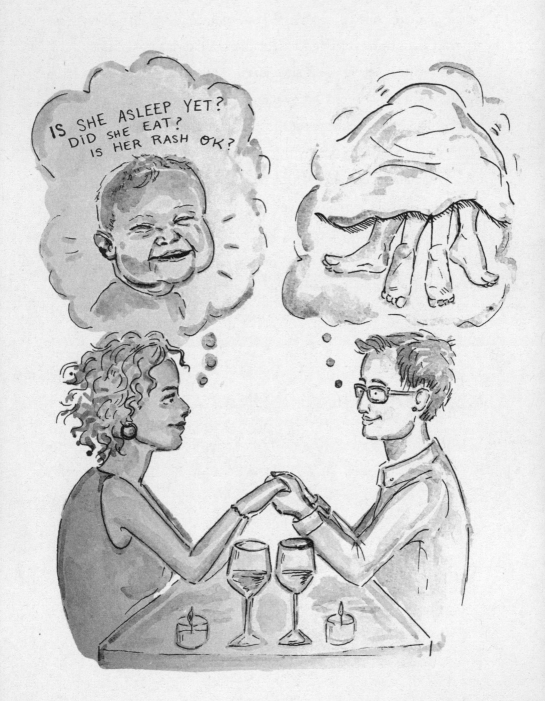

The First Year of Motherhood

Your Baby, Her Own Person

When you gave birth, you experienced a profound separation from your baby, who had, until then, existed only inside your body. Suddenly, she was her own creature, out in the world. Now, as she grows and develops from a squirming newborn into an actual person, one of your primary tasks is to learn how to see her as an individual. Even in her first year, her successes (the first time she pulls herself up to standing) and struggles (the first time she purses her lips and refuses to eat any food) are hers, not yours. The foundation for a psychologically healthy parent-child relationship is set when you learn this lesson: You don't get to control what your baby wants, needs, or ultimately does. That does not mean that you aren't the parent in charge, it just means that the dance of your relationship will involve improvising and alternating who takes the lead.

By now you will have passed through many of your "firsts," and you and the baby may be able to establish a routine. You'll be able to spend more time venturing out of the house with your child, and part of your matrescence journey will be a discovery of how the world reacts to you both. Be prepared for compliments ("She's as adorable as her mother!"), complicated compliments ("That's a she? Well, she looks like a sweet little baby boy!"), criticism ("You really shouldn't be bringing him out without a hat"), comparison ("Isn't he small for an eight-month-old?"), and the irrational praise of baby-exceptionalism ("I can already see that she's a genius by the look in her eyes").

Your baby is her own person, and you are your own woman. Even the most confident and secure mother will sometimes feel rattled by a stranger's comments. The more you can keep your gaze on the relationship between the two of you and avoid looking at others for validation, the better a parent you will be, and the more secure your child will eventually become. The same advice goes for accepting and supporting the individuality of your relationship with your partner, as well as the specificity of his relationship with the baby.

When you're struggling with a parenting question or your child is going through a challenging phase, try not to think of these moments as "problems." We've introduced the concept of a good enough mother, and from now on (and, really, forever), we want to encourage you to think about accepting your baby as a good enough child.

Try not to become preoccupied with goals. Weight and height growth charts, as well as other development milestones you may read about, are basically markers created for doctors to track a baby's development and intervene if any health issues arise. But these numbers, from your baby's birth weight to the other percentiles, are not a score of how well you're doing as a caretaker.

If your baby is in the thirtieth percentile on the growth chart and your pediatrician says everything is okay, believe her. If your gut is telling you that something is wrong, then ask for a second opinion. But if your friend's baby is in the ninetieth percentile, that doesn't mean her baby is healthier or that she's a better mother or doing something you should try. It probably just means that everyone in her family is tall. Healthy babies come in all shapes and sizes, so do your best to view your child's growth through an individual lens.

Attachment

Attunement, Temperament, and Goodness of Fit

"Attachment" is the term psychologists use to describe how babies and their caretakers bond. One way to think about attachment is from the perspective of evolutionary biology—since babies are exhausting, nature has designed them to be adorable so we're inspired to care for them. But we don't bond with our babies just because they're beautiful. There's the mysterious ingredient of love—and the physical influence of oxytocin, one of the hormones released during pregnancy and around childbirth. Breastfeeding and skin-to-skin touch also help to get the attachment chemicals flowing.

Studies have shown that a baby's need for affection may be even more powerful than his need for physical nurturing. In the 1950s, psychologist Harry Harlow studied newborn rhesus monkeys, giving them food and shelter but no cuddly mother figure—they had only a wire food dispenser that provided no physical comfort. When Harlow compared this group to another group of monkeys who were underfed but had the physical nurturing of a soft, fluffy object in their crib, he saw that the second group of babies grew up to have healthier behaviors and were much better at calming down from stress. This research is one of the foundational works of attachment theory—it shows that emotional bonding is just as important for healthy development as food, water, and the biological "necessities" of life.

Laying the groundwork for a healthy attachment in infancy is one of the most important things you can do to set your child on a path of lifelong emotional wellness. However, attachment does not follow a formula. While abuse and neglect will damage any baby, a "good enough" attachment can be formed in many different ways.

Psychologists who study mother-infant attachment often talk about the quality of "attunement," which is the way a mother and baby communicate nonverbally so that the caretaker is able to pick up on the baby's needs through facial expressions and other gestures.

In the first few months, most of your communication will be accomplished via facial expressions. In the 1970s, psychologist Edward Tronick's "Still Face" experiment showed how strongly babies respond to their mother's nonverbal communications. Babies have an innate need to communicate, to see and be seen, months before they learn to speak or can understand spoken language. **Your baby can't read your mind, but in a way, he can read your face.** And, as anyone who has ever been able to tell that someone is lying by the look in his eyes can tell you, the micro-movements of our face reveal our emotions. So, a mother's emotional state (which will impact the animation of her facial expressions and the warmth of her physical affection) is as essential for her child's growth as milk.

Attachment is a two-way street. You may not think that such a tiny human could have a personality or "self." But psychological studies of a human characteristic called "temperament" suggest that babies may be born with a personality or emotional style. Both nature and nurture will shape how your child grows over time, but some qualities, like sensitivity to noise, shyness, and even sense of humor, may be as programmed in his genes as his height.

In the 1960s, psychologists Alexander Thomas, Stella Chess, and Herbert Birch created a rubric to organize a baby's temperament into one of three basic groups: easy, difficult, and slow to warm up.

Easy babies are generally in a pleasant mood, good sleepers, and readily adaptable to changes in their environment, such as trying new foods and adjusting to sleeping in a new room. Difficult babies tend to be fussy and challenging to soothe. They are more sensitive to disruptions in their routine, and even with a regular schedule, they may have more trouble falling into a rhythm with their sleeping and eating patterns, as if their biological clocks are harder to set. Slow-to-warm-up babies are cautious around new situations and people, but when they become familiar with a new environment or new schedule, they can be as adaptable as easy babies.

Within and between these three categories, babies vary in their personalities almost as much as adults do. Ask any mother with more than one child, and she'll tell you how each baby made her distinct personality known. Some are active wiggle worms, and others prefer to hang out and rest. Some are flirty with strangers, and others are shy. Some babies are intensely expressive—when they're happy or sad or hungry, they make sure you know it loud and clear—and others are harder to read.

Just as every baby has a temperament, so does every mother. "Goodness of fit" describes the match between a baby's temperament and her mother's. Sometimes the fit is complementary: a relaxed, low-key mother and an easy baby, for example. That same relaxed mother might also have a complementary fit with a difficult baby who is hard to soothe and requires a lot of patience. The point of goodness of fit is not that the mother and baby need to have the same personality style, but that understanding where your two personalities mesh or clash can be helpful as your relationship unfolds.

Some mothers and babies struggle with their goodness of fit. If you crave physical closeness, you may feel rejected if your baby wriggles away from you when you want to cuddle. If you're not very energetic, you may find an exuberant baby overwhelming. As one of our patients who was more sensitive to noise described: "At first I used to find being in the same room with the baby to be grating— his squeals and crying were so loud, and I just wanted to turn down the volume! But eventually I learned he just had a big personality. I'm still grateful for peace and quiet at the end of the day after he's sleeping, but I'm getting used to it. Even if he hurts my ears, it doesn't shock or worry me anymore, and now I just associate it with how much I love having him around."

If many interactions with your baby feel like a power struggle, it may be a sign that you're experiencing a temperamental mismatch. This can be exhausting and demoralizing, and it's a good idea to ask for help—from your partner, your parents or in-laws, child care workers, or your pediatrician or other health care providers. They may have different suggestions for how to soothe the baby, or they may pitch in to give you a break. It's smart to expand your supports. And sometimes you can find a quick fix. Many of our patients initially thought the problem was with the bond between them and their baby, but when they described the issue to the pediatrician, she helped them identify a medical issue like gastric reflux. As soon as they found the right treatment, the baby was much less fussy and more able to enjoy his mother's affection.

What to Do If You're Not a "Good Fit"

If you and your baby have a difficult fit, it can be hard not to take the struggle personally. One of our patients said: "When I try to burp the baby, he seems to scream even harder. It's like he knows that I don't have maternal instincts." Another said, "Whenever I put her down for a nap, she spits up and I need to change her whole outfit—it's like she's trying to torture me."

If you find these kinds of thoughts looping through your head, you may be experiencing a distortion that psychologists call "personalization." It's when you take things personally when they are not really about you. Infants are not sophisticated enough to intentionally manipulate your feelings. If you feel like they are pulling your puppet strings, they're probably just communicating that they are hungry, uncomfortable, wet, scared, or wanting to be held. If you're feeling particularly resentful at your baby for "rejecting you" or "torturing you," you may want to spend some time journaling or talking to a friend or therapist. You may find some connection to other difficult relationships from your past that left you feeling unlovable, and realize that you're projecting this past pain onto your baby's communications. In our experience, talking about the residual pain can help you learn how to take your baby's communications less personally.

Another approach is to try a mindfulness mantra. Write down some centering statements to remind you that no matter how frustrated you feel, your baby is just a baby, and mothering is sometimes simply this hard. You can read these truths whenever you are feeling on edge. Here are some examples that have been helpful for our patients:

- He is who he is, and he'd probably be crying with any mother.
- I have checked everything that I could fix (hunger/diaper/sleep/ etc.) and there's nothing else I can do. I'm not the cause of his distress.
- Sometimes parents can't make discomfort go away, and when I show him that I can handle his being upset, it's good for our long-term relationship. I love him no matter what.
- The pediatrician said his behavior is normal and I shouldn't worry.
- My job is to watch to see if there's a pattern to his crying rather than panicking.
- This happens sometimes, and it doesn't last forever. If I can be patient, this too shall pass.
- It's okay to walk away for a minute and give myself a break if he's crying but safe in his crib. If I'm feeling too angry or intolerant, maybe I need something to eat, to go to the bathroom, or simply to get two minutes of quiet.

Psychologist Beatrice Beebe studied mother-baby relationships by analyzing videotaped sessions of mothers interacting with their babies. Freeze-frames on the images showed that when there is a complementary match, a mother and child might simultaneously move toward and away from each other, as in a dance. For example, if a baby is feeling overwhelmed by the mother's attempts to feed him and looks away, a complementary response from the mother would be to sit back, give him some space, and wait for him to look at her again to reengage.

One way to think about this research is that your baby will teach you how to parent her. She will get your attention when she needs you, and push you away when she's ready to explore, foster independence, or calm herself down. We encourage all parents to trust what feels right to them when it comes to early parenting. **As we often remind our patients: Do your best not to get in their way, and your child will show you the way.**

There's No Perfect Attachment

When we talk about attachment, many parents think of "attachment parenting." This is a parenting philosophy that encourages continuous physical contact with the baby. While there are many benefits of skin-to-skin touch, science hasn't shown that physical contact needs to be 24/7 constant for your baby's well-being.

Most of the parenting advice in this book reflects our professional perspective: There is more than one psychologically

healthy way to raise a child. We recommend that you follow your heart and your gut.

Psychoanalyst John Bowlby was one of the early researchers of attachment theory. He believed that a baby's attachment to his primary caretakers creates a prototype, an "internal working model," upon which the child's future relationships will be built. Bowlby believed that this model becomes the foundation of the persons's self-esteem and gives him the sense of how trustworthy other people are. Research on how childhood attachment informs adult relationships has continued to develop and advance since Bowlby's work in the mid–twentieth century, but we still agree with his basic tenet: The way we bond with our parents is an important framework for how we learn to love.

There is some scientific debate over how much of a child's attachment style is nature and how much is nurture. So, as with many dimensions of parenting, the style of your child's attachment may be somewhat out of your control. However, there are some general principles of development that may help you to better understand when and why your child is behaving in a way that is more tentative, clingy, or adventurous.

Psychoanalyst Margaret Mahler theorized that early on, a baby is in a "symbiotic" phase with his mother. In the first few months of life, he experiences himself and his mother as one entity, perhaps even thinking that they are one person. Sometime after five months, the baby begins "separation-individuation," an early awareness that his mother is a separate person. "Practicing" comes next, when a baby is physically able to crawl, then walk, and becomes more interested in exploring the outside world.

As a baby learns how to crawl and then walk away from his mom, he will begin to check in with her, sometimes by looking back for reassurance. This is called "rapprochement" behavior, which also involves returning to the mother's side at intervals after adventuring away.

Some theories suggest that how a mother manages her baby's separation and reunion may influence his attachment style as an adult. Psychologist Mary Ainsworth theorized that a child with "secure attachment" experiences his mother as a safe home base; he can leave her side because he is confident that she will be there when he returns.

Healthy attachment isn't about a mother and child being physically attached to each other at all times but, rather, the result of the child's sense of security in being loved and cared for. Therefore, if you're a mom who works outside the home and is away from your baby often, there is no reason to suspect that attachment problems will arise as long as whoever is taking care of him makes him feel as loved as you do. **A baby can develop secure attachment even if she has multiple alternating caretakers.** If everyone who cares for her makes her feel safe, she will learn that relationships are reliable, trustworthy, nurturing, and supportive.

Sleep Training

A baby's sleep and feeding patterns will shift during the first year as her brain matures. Generally, as they get older, babies develop the ability to sleep through the night. "Sleep training" is a term with varying definitions. In general, it refers to techniques that parents can attempt to encourage their babies to sleep through the night as independently as possible. Some popular elements of sleep training include: a consistent bedtime routine; putting your baby down to sleep while he is still awake (rather than rocking him to sleep in your arms); and "crying it out," which generally means leaving your baby alone (for some amount of time) if he cries at night, instead of rushing to pick him up to soothe him yourself.

We believe that there is no singular "right" way to approach sleep training with your baby, and pediatricians, child care experts, and parents may offer you a range of differing opinions (see **Resources**). Some may suggest that you not try to sleep train at all, but let your child organically learn how to sleep through the night.

Many pediatricians recommend trying the "Five S's" approach to soothe crying babies described by Harvey Karp, MD, in his book *The Happiest Baby on the Block*. Other guides recommend that parents establish a consistent pre-bedtime ritual (bathing, feeding, rocking, and singing are some common approaches) and then put the baby down to sleep while he is still awake. Parents are advised to leave the baby alone, even if he cries—initially for short periods of time and then, on future nights, for longer. The theory is that this gradual technique teaches the baby, eventually, to be able to sleep on his own.

There are many different sleep training methods; each has its different particular recommendations, and there have been many modern revisions (see **Resources** and **References**), so think about what will be best for your baby's temperament and your own.

If you choose to use a "cry it out" method, discuss with your pediatrician if, and at what age, this might be appropriate for your baby. Hearing your baby cry at night can be distressing, but when done appropriately under your doctor's instructions it is not harmful. Being disciplined while training your baby to sleep doesn't mean that you have to stop all the affectionate and playful activities you and your baby enjoy during the day; you won't always have to be bad cop.

Most parents find that sleep training requires several attempts, or at least reinforcements at different times in a baby's development. Teething, travel, a new room, and transitioning from a bassinette to a crib are just a few of the common triggers that may cause babies to regress in their sleep patterns. This means that another round of sleep training may be required before they are once again able to sleep on their own.

If you'd like to train your baby to sleep (or at least to benefit from the successful results) but you're reluctant because you're worried that it will hurt your baby, your pediatrician may be able to offer you reassurance about the healthy parameters for leaving a crying baby alone at night. If your baby is healthy and mature enough that her doctor is recommending the training, that means that she will likely benefit from it and also be able to tolerate the associated minor discomforts, like a wet diaper that you might find in the morning.

Many pediatricians do not endorse any one particular method but suggest that you consider a behavioral approach (meaning, some kind of sleep training) to help your baby develop healthy sleep patterns. In general, it is thought that children benefit from eventually learning how to fall asleep without requiring their parent's physical touch, a skill related to "self-soothing."

Self-soothing is the foundation for a person's ability to calm herself down, and it often sets the stage for healthy adult patterns. The ability to relax your mind and your body, without requiring the help of another person or a crutch like alcohol or food, is a good habit to develop early. Many professionals who strongly advocate sleep training have this long-term concern in mind.

Some parents who struggle with sleep training for their children may have a history of their own difficulties with self-soothing. Many of us have our own fraught experiences with bedtime, either from adult insomnia or from memories of our own childhood fears in the dark. We may bring this anxiety to our decision-making about how to parent. One of our patients was motivated to train her baby to sleep, but found that her daughter's cries were intensely distressing. She came in to her therapy appointment confused about her dramatic response. In therapy, this patient realized she was connecting her daughter's distress to her own bedtime anxiety. She said, "Every Sunday night, I get so anxious about going back to work, I lie in bed for hours without falling asleep. I have my own feelings of dread about insomnia, and realized that I was extra-sensitive to my daughter's nighttime issues because I was stressed-out myself about getting enough sleep." This patient found it helpful to ask her husband to take over sleep training while she put in headphones to listen to soothing music and block out the baby's cries, trusting that he would take care of the baby so that she could focus on winding down.

Another patient came in to address her guilt for feeling so "cold" in the face of her daughter's sleep-training cries. She said it was as if her emotions completely shut off when her daughter cried from her crib. This turned out to have its roots in her own history of childhood trauma. This patient said, "Growing up, I shared a room with my three younger siblings, and my parents weren't very attentive. When the two littlest ones were a toddler and a baby, I remember lying in bed while they were crying. It was awful." She'd had to shut down her emotional response to the sound of a child's cries before, and this memory was triggered when she listened to her own baby's cries, along with the feeling of numbness that she used in childhood to distance herself emotionally.

This mother was helped by learning that even though she felt numb when her baby cried, that had nothing to do with her love for her child. She was able to be emotionally present in other ways, empathic and responsive to her child's feelings, and given her healthy attachment with the baby, this was clearly "good enough" to provide for a nurturing emotional environment. She gave herself permission to continue to be someone who needs some emotional space around other people when they're crying in distress, and she was able to let go of some of these feelings of guilt.

 ## How to Cope If Sleep Training Makes You Cry

- **If you feel guilty that you're not more guilty:** Some of our patients tell us that they feel ashamed if they don't experience "crying-it-out" as gut-wrenching. If you can tolerate your baby's crying, don't be alarmed. You may simply appreciate that this approach is helping him learn how to become more independent, not hurting him. Everyone benefits when you can sleep through the night.

- **If your pain feels like too much:** For some parents, separating from a tearful baby at night triggers their own anxiety about separation, loss, or trauma from a different time in their life. If you feel your heart pounding or fear and anger rising while you're training your baby, you may need to slow down or change your approach. Journaling or talking about how the experience makes you feel may help connect some dots of what's triggered inside you by your baby's crying.

- **Ask for help and take breaks:** Maybe you will realize over time that sleep training is not right for you, and that you and your baby will work on your approach to bedtime in another way.

Or maybe once you're calm and have a chance to reflect, you'll decide that your baby is benefiting by learning how to sleep for longer intervals. If you have a partner, ask her to take over. If you're alone, then maybe give yourself a break, soothe the baby until you feel calmer, and remind yourself that you can just try again tomorrow. Take some deep breaths, take a hot bath, or do whatever feels soothing to calm your nervous system.

- **Try these mantras:** Remind yourself that you and your baby are safe. Tears are just tears; they don't cause any permanent damage. Remind yourself that teaching a baby how to self-soothe in healthy, appropriate intervals, while providing plenty of comfort throughout the day, is not the same thing as abuse or neglect. Remember that this is a stage of parenting that almost everyone finds stressful. Know that it's okay to have no idea what approach is best for you and your family. There are many more nights to work on this, and you can always change your mind or try again. As with other milestones, we encourage you not to think in terms of success and failure (especially on your first night of sleep training).

- **And if you still don't feel better:** If you can't calm yourself down, are worried about how angry and frustrated you're feeling toward your baby, or just would like more support, we encourage you to call your pediatrician, doctor, or a mental health professional and talk about what's going on.

How you decide to sleep train your baby will depend on his temperament and yours, as well as your personal parenting philosophy. Also, your own personal life circumstances or schedule may guide what feels best to you. Many of our patients who work nights doing shift work, or have to travel for work, enjoy the continued nighttime contact through feeding or cuddling with their babies, so they may have their own preferences for how to sleep train (or not).

The Adventure of Solid Foods

Just as soon as you feel like you've settled into a good place with feeding your baby milk or formula, it's time to figure out the solid foods. This is likely to be another one of those exciting and anxiety-producing "firsts."

Parents may experience great pleasure in watching their children enjoy the new sensations of eating: the squish of avocado between their fingers and the tang of mango on their tongue. But alongside this excitement, it's natural to have thoughts of worry that your child may choke or have an allergic reaction. You may fear that if your baby prefers sweeter foods to vegetables, that will start a lifetime of bad habits. Some babies will have periods of time when they refuse to eat or will eat only if they can feed themselves—a slow and messy process that adds a new layer of stress to the situation.

There are very few things that a baby can do on his own, and early on, eating is one of the firsts. The more a child connects eating with struggles around discipline and control, the more his relationship to food may eventually become a communication about power. Changes in eating behavior are sometimes not about food at all but simply a way your baby is learning. Developmentally speaking, if your baby is (temporarily) being stubborn about eating, this might even be a good thing if it shows a healthy exploration of independence and agency. Consider letting him play out his willful experiments, or lead the way by feeding himself, and he may likely return to his normal eating patterns.

As with other parenting questions, if you're not sure how to handle a certain change in eating behaviors, your first call should be to the pediatrician. If your baby's growth is not a concern, many pediatricians will advise parents to follow their child's lead rather than aggressively intervene. Healthy babies will generally eat when they're hungry and slow down when their growth demands are lower. Many doctors advise that as long as your child is healthy, you shouldn't push too hard to change her idiosyncratic eating preferences.

As your baby is figuring out her relationship to food, she will also feel your influence. When you became a parent, you already had a lifetime of your own relationship to eating. Your feelings about what and how much your baby eats will be shaped by your own history. Did your parents put pressure on you and insist you clean your plate? Was your mother always worried about getting fat, and did she scold you if you served yourself seconds?

Your baby, guided by instinct and desire, is not born with any rules or ideas about eating. Be mindful of what habits, beliefs, and values you do and don't want to pass on to her. The best way to do this is by being aware of what your own issues are. Are there foods you fear eating because you see them as "bad" or because you can't control yourself once you start eating them? Do you count calories and berate yourself when you make a "mistake"? Pay attention to your emotional response to your baby's food exploration, and rather than reacting in the moment—scolding her for making a mess or wasting food, or refusing to give her seconds—note your reaction and reflect on it later. You can't prevent your feelings, but you can avoid passing down your hang-ups.

One of our patients told us, "I've always struggled with my weight, and I wanted my daughter to just be happy with her body and to be able to enjoy food. But as soon as she started eating solid foods, I found myself pushing her to eat greens and protein, and feeling like I'd failed when I gave her those processed puffs. My friend pointed out that allowing her to explore might not cause unhealthy patterns, but being too strict about rules actually might, because when you make some foods forbidden, that's when kids start seeing them as special."

Because our emotional patterns around food can be so deeply ingrained, many of us are unsure how to identify them, let alone avoid passing them on to our children. If you'd like to learn more, consider exploring some of the **Resources** for this chapter to find different professional perspectives on the early years of feeding.

The Psychology of Weaning

When babies are weaned, either from breast milk to formula or from breast milk to solid foods, complicated feelings may arise. Stopping breastfeeding triggers a chemical change in your body: Your oxytocin and prolactin levels fall, and your periods may return if they haven't already. All these fluctuations may impact your mood (especially if you have been emotionally sensitive to other hormonal shifts, such as around pregnancy and postpartum or around your menstrual cycle).

Some women find weaning a relief. Your body is finally yours again. You don't have to coordinate regular intervals or strict hours when you can leave the house (or have to bring your pump). But many of our patients who found breastfeeding to be physically uncomfortable or emotionally stressful tell us that they fear judgment for no longer breastfeeding, or they feel guilty when they choose to wean, like they're putting their own desires above their baby's needs. One of our patients feared that if she stopped breastfeeding, she would feel less confident about her role in taking care of her daughter: "My husband and mom play with her and make her laugh around bath time. They're great at feeding her solids. I'm the only one who breastfeeds and gives her that comfort. After I wean, what am I really going to offer that's so special?"

The guilt generally subsides after weaning when you can observe that your baby is doing just fine, in terms of feeding, comfort, weight gain, and their love for you. Weaning isn't likely to impact your attachment in any long-term way. The bonding time that you used to spend with your baby breastfeeding will be transferred to other activities. And weaning may benefit your energy—if you're less physically depleted, you may find that you're able to be more patient and playful with the baby.

If you enjoyed nursing but have to wean against your wishes, for medical reasons, because of issues with breastfeeding/pumping, or due to any other undesired situation, you may grieve the experience. Some women come to us in tears, without having connected these tender emotions to their weaning process. Others know that their sadness is tied to the weaning because it's connected to something larger. As one of our patients described, "I'm sad because he's not a baby anymore. He doesn't fit into those sweet little newborn clothes. And we don't have that bonding time during feedings. I'll never have time with him like that again."

The experience of weaning is symbolic of the many separations to come. Childbirth is the baby's first separation from your body; no longer feeding from your breast may be considered the second. These sentimental, bittersweet transitions can be viewed as symbolic about the circle of life. Of course, all parents want their children to grow up healthy and strong. But with every milestone comes another inch forward in a child growing up and away from being dependent on you. After your baby first crawls and then walks, he needs you less for mobility. In potty training, she no longer needs you to change her diaper. Alongside your joy, it's not uncommon to also have some feelings of mourning around your child's development because it also represents the passage of time.

Is "Mommy Brain" a Real Thing?

Many women feel like pregnancy and early motherhood "does something" to their brain. In the first months after birth, you may feel foggy and slow, like you've lost the ability to find the right words when having a "grown-up" conversation. You may get your baby to sleep and then step into the shower without taking off your glasses. You finally make time for a phone call to connect with a good friend, and catch yourself nodding off in the middle of the conversation.

While "mommy brain" might sound like a misogynist myth, it's not necessarily a deficiency—it's the result of a host of changes to your body, brain, and emotions. With so much changing in your life, it's natural that your brain would adapt.

Science has a long way to go in understanding how growing, delivering, and even feeding and parenting a baby may influence a woman's brain, but research has shown that the biological impact is real. Whether it's from sleep deprivation or hormones, some pregnant women and new mothers struggle with a specific type of memory involved in recalling small details such as specific words, like the name of a restaurant. However, there is no convincing scientific evidence that pregnancy or motherhood makes you any less smart.

It may be that some aspects of memory are sacrificed to enhance others. Some studies have shown that pregnancy instigates brain changes in regions involved in social cognition or empathy. One

theory is that these changes may have an evolutionary benefi
strengthen the communication between a mother and her in:
sharpening your ability to pick up on your baby's nonve
communication through facial expressions and cries.

In the 1950s, decades before scientists started using functi
neuroimaging to study changes in brain activity, the psychoana
Donald Winnicott—of the good enough mother—publishe
paper titled "Primary Maternal Preoccupation." In it he descri
the intense psychological demands of taking care of a creatur
helpless and dependent as a newborn.

It's hard to pay attention, emotionally and cognitively, to y
baby and yourself at the same time. This can be complicated
the guilt many of our patients tell us that they feel when they s
their attention to themselves. As one of our patients described: '
like I'm never paying attention to any one thing. Like I'm ne
fully listening or present. When I'm at my desk, I'm thinking ab
what I want to do with the baby that weekend, and when I'm ho
with her, I'm thinking about the presentation I have to prepare
work. I feel like crap because sometimes I feel like nothing's do
well." In fact, this woman was doing great at her job and was als
wonderful mother. But like many new mothers, these new demar
of multitasking made her doubt herself.

Many new mothers tell us that they find themselves feeli
like their mind is never in one place. We hear this so often th
we've given this experience its own name, "the divided mind." V
think of the divided mind as a cognitive and emotional state th

is a consequence of the changes in how you spend your time and attention when growing and then caring for a totally dependent human being. **Your mind is literally divided, as you're dealing with your own life while tending to another's.**

Perhaps the best way to explain this phenomenon is to think of your mind as a superhighway. In this analogy, think of being unpartnered as driving on a one-lane road. On this road, you have to keep to the speed limit and pay attention to the traffic signs in order to drive safely, but the demands on your attention are straightforward.

When you share your life with a partner, the interpersonal demands may put you on a two-lane freeway. One lane is your life, the second lane your partner's. There are signs on both sides of the road, and they may lead you in different directions. Decisions—as big as whether or not you're going to move or as small as what you're going to have for dinner—now require a conversation or negotiation with another person. Driving requires more cognitive and emotional effort.

When you're pregnant, you've merged onto a highway with three lanes, minimum. You're managing doctors' appointments, the needs of your changing body, and new feelings of excitement and worry. You're also processing your thoughts and conflicting demands like *"All I want to do is take a nap, but I also want to meet my friend for brunch."*

After the baby arrives, her full-time needs require full-time attention. When you're sitting with her on the play mat, your mind may be divided by other tasks for her (*"Do we have enough diapers*

in the house?"), other tasks for you ("*It would be nice to take a shower today*"), and your other responsibilities and relationships ("*I really should return that email*"). Many mothers tell us that even when their partner or someone else is taking care of the baby, their own mental "lane" of awareness of the baby's needs continues to be active. As one patient described, "Even when I'm at work, a part of me is also thinking: *What is she doing right now?* I'm still able to do my job, but now it's like I have two jobs, and when I'm at work I also miss her. When I'm home, I also find myself thinking about work, and want to get back to this project I'm excited about. I wanted to go to my friend's bachelorette party, but all night I kept looking at photos of my baby. I'm just all over the place."

Another way to think of mommy brain is that it's a little like having jet lag. Sleep deprivation plays a significant role. Have you ever taken a trip across time zones and tried to get work done the day you return? It usually doesn't go as well as you'd hoped. Shuttling between being out in the world with other adults and home with the baby can feel like you're traveling between two different worlds, emotionally and behaviorally. The disruption to your sleep (the amount, exposure to sunlight, and when sleep occurs), less recreation and rest, and irregular mealtimes are disorienting on their own, without factoring in all your new responsibilities and the hormonal and emotional shifts.

That being said, there is no universal experience of mommy brain. Just as every woman's menstrual or pregnancy experience is different, no single rule dictates how every woman's brain and emotions will respond to hormones and life changes. And mothers with different personalities, lifestyles, personal demands, and family structures may experience this adjustment differently. We believe that more studies need to be done to learn about brain changes during pregnancy and parenting, taking into account the hormonal shifts as well as associated changes in behavior and emotions.

Returning to Work or Stay-at-Home Mothering

Most new mothers tell us that matrescence involves a change in their workplace identities. Unfortunately, this change often brings a struggle. It seems as if the cultural conversation of work and motherhood are moving forward, but frankly, in the U.S. especially, it's still a big mess, with unaffordable child care and workplace traditions that penalize mothers and interfere with their advancement. It's difficult for two working parents to share the load if they don't have equal benefits and opportunities at work. As American society continues to be largely unaccommodating to the demands of working parents, families have to answer tough personal questions about their finances, child care options and philosophies, and the division of labor between partners.

Most women, especially single moms, cannot afford to quit their jobs outside of the home. But some women may consider the option of being a stay-at-home mom (SAHM) if they do the math and compare the expense of child care to their salary and decide that their job isn't extrinsically or intrinsically valuable enough to continue. Other parents decide to stay at home because they find the work of child care to be more rewarding than their prior job, or they feel strongly about the personal value of stay-at-home parenting. And of course, there are many other scenarios, including parents who work in paying jobs from home, work part-time, and those who are at home because they cannot find employment despite needing a paying job.

In addition to financial questions, we recommend that you also think about how your work factors into your identity: How much does your job make you tick? Do you feel most like yourself at home, or do you thrive being out and about, not only working, but also coming to and from work, and from the associated routine and adult interaction? If you're considering leaving your job, we recommend you consider how this change will impact your sense of meaning, productivity, independence, and community.

Some women tell us that they find these questions overwhelming because, in their twenties and thirties (the time when many are having children), they may be still figuring out their professional identities. They may know they want to be mothers, but they may not have found their dream job, so it's hard to assess how work factors into their sense of self. It's confusing to try to negotiate all of these choices simultaneously when so many parts of your life are still in flux.

We encourage you to try to make your decisions about work and motherhood based on what you *want*, not based on what you *fear*. Try to remember that you can change your mind down the road, and that ambivalence is natural with life transitions, and certainly in new motherhood.

As much as you may plan in advance, many of our patients tell us that it was hard to predict what being a SAHM or going back to work would feel like. You can't know if you'll like taking care of your baby seven days a week, or how the workday separation from her will feel, until you try it out. We know stay-at-home moms who missed not only the income but the routine, stimulation, and adult interaction of office work. We know "career women" who surprised themselves by deciding to take a longer leave or to quit their jobs altogether. And we know women who were on the fence and were surprised to find their careers blooming after motherhood, or found themselves benefiting from a productive professional change or interpersonal skills strengthened by motherhood.

One of our patients who decided to shorten her maternity leave and go back to work early shared this story: "The dirty little secret of motherhood is that sometimes it's easier when you're back at work. Even though you have more to do in the day, for me, it actually felt like there was more time to get things done. By the time I got home, I always felt more connected to my kids because I missed them, rather than feeling sick of them. Your work routine adds order and predictability to everything in your life—it's so much harder to control your schedule when you're at home."

Another patient who was a SAHM told us, "My job didn't give me a paid maternity leave, and since our families lived far away and we couldn't afford to hire anyone, I had to quit my job and stay at home. Honestly, I think it was helpful not to have the choice, because I would have had a hard time making the decision. I tried to see it as a blessing in disguise, and it really was. I enjoyed spending every day with my baby, and I ended up meeting some other moms in the neighborhood who are now my best friends. It's sort of like having coworkers—we meet and give each other advice and do clothing swaps. It's really nice."

When they're pondering staying home vs. returning to work, many women worry about external judgment more than their own well-being. Mothers who consider staying at home may worry about being criticized by others (even and especially other moms) for what they're "giving up," being seen as "boring," "*just* a mom," or "not strong enough" to manage the juggling act. If you're going back to work, you may fear being judged as someone who "values her career more than her family," or who is "less invested" in her child's day-to-day wellness than a SAHM.

You may also feel pressure because of the choices your mother and other women in your family made: "She regretted giving up her career, so I'm not going to" or "I hated coming home from school when she was still at work, so I'm going to quit my job." It's important to remember that no matter how strongly you feel about your mother's choices, and no matter how much you have in common, you're a different person in a different generation. Beware of making a reactionary decision based on what did or didn't work for your mother and her circumstances rather than your own.

If you're struggling with judgment from your mother or other family members about your plans, we encourage you to discuss your situation with your partner and trusted friends. One of our patients shared this story: "My mother-in-law was so judgmental when I went back to work. She's the queen of passive-aggressive digs. One day I finally lost my patience when she said, 'You do know what happens to children who go to day care?' I replied, 'YES. They turn out just as well as children of stay-at-home moms—maybe even better, because everyone gets some breathing room!'"

While this patient was glad that she defended herself, she also regretted letting her frustration simmer and explode into an angry confrontation. After she was able to process her own conflicted feelings about missing some experiences with her kids because she was at work, she was able to have a productive talk with her husband about how her mother-in-law was making her feel. This didn't necessarily change the mother-in-law's personality, but it helped our patient feel more supported by her husband.

Returning to work after maternity leave is demanding, both logistically and emotionally. You may be looking forward to returning to work but sad to leave your baby. You may be dreading the pile on your desk and in your email in-box, or you may be a little disappointed that your colleagues so seamlessly moved on without you. You may feel newly motivated professionally after some time away, but nervous about your ability to keep up with your colleagues. You may feel fine once you've settled into your workday, and on the weekends when you're home and reconnected with your baby for longer stretches of time, but find the transitions in between the two modes and their separations exhausting.

One of our patients described the most difficult part of returning to work as the transition between work and home: "The first few weeks back at work were hard, but not in the ways I had expected. I was okay in terms of missing my baby, and I didn't worry about him during the day. But then I'd get home and feel like I had no idea what I was doing. I felt like his babysitter rather than his mom, which made me feel resentful—of my job, for keeping me away; and of my baby, for becoming this creature I didn't know how to take care of anymore."

The feeling of disconnection was partly because she was in "another mode at work," but also because she felt that she didn't have enough information about the baby's day to make good choices for him at night. She realized that the distance between her two roles—at work and at home—could be bridged with information. She started asking her son's babysitter for more updates during the day and a detailed debrief when she got home. (She also explained to the babysitter why she wanted this extra information and that it wasn't about micromanaging.) "I had a list of things I wanted to know, like how much time they had been out of the house. Little things like how wound up or tuckered out he had been during the day helped me make better sense of how he was behaving at night when I got home." For this mom, learning about the minutiae of her son's life helped her feel more confident in her instincts with him after the handoff.

Easing Back In

Many mothers tell us that their anxiety peaks in the weeks leading up to their return to work (in fact, this is one of the most common times for women to call us for help). Even if you know that your baby is safe with a trustworthy caretaker, the physical experience of separation may set off evolutionary alarm bells that take some time to quiet down.

If you're worried that your baby will not be able to thrive in your absence, you will likely be reassured once you get into your new routine and see that you're both absolutely fine—sometimes even better! But whether you're anxious about being away from your baby or anxious about readjusting to work, this transition, like most big changes, can be challenging.

If possible, we recommend returning to work gradually. This will help you process all of these different emotions and figure out your new routine at a slightly slower pace. At the very least, see if you can make your first week back shorter by starting on a Wednesday or Thursday; consider asking about working shorter days at first or part-time for a while. Find out if your job allows telecommuting. And if there isn't a standard for any of these approaches for moms returning from maternity leave, see if you can request one.

If you're able to arrange for a slower return, you can ease your child into day care or start your babysitter, nanny, or family member who will be helping part-time. You can leave extra time for organizing, rest, and managing the new logistics of commuting, pumping, and adjusting to life as a working mom. It's a big adjustment.

Depending on where you work, you may already have clear boundaries between your work and home life. But if you're used to being available to your job 24/7, you may need to discuss new off-hours, or how to reach you in case of a true emergency, and to explain that there may be a delay in other after-hours correspondence.

When you return to your job, your colleagues and boss may welcome you back warmly, or you may sense (accurately or not) an undercurrent of tension because they perceive that you've been "off" while they have been carrying the load. **We don't need to tell you that our society has a long way to go in creating work cultures that are more accommodating to parents.** We recommend our **Resources** and books cited to help educate you about your rights and to help you advocate for yourself.

CBT for the Gray Zones of Work/Life Balance

As we've described for other aspects of matrescence, figuring out your work/life balance presents many challenging dilemmas with no right answers. When faced with these kinds of decisions, many people try to oversimplify their choices. This can provide some relief and reassurance that you're making a "good" choice, even if it's an arbitrary binary. But it can also leave you with the added burden of fearing a "bad" choice, when most of these decisions will fall in a gray zone that naturally stirs up feelings of ambivalence.

Here are some examples of how to reframe black-and-white thinking around back-to-work dilemmas:

- **Black-and-white:** "Going back to work isn't worth missing my baby's first steps."

    Flexible: "Yes, I may miss those first steps if I'm at work, or if I'm in the bathroom and the baby is exploring in her playpen. Since I'm with her every day, I'll probably be there at some point on the first day she makes a new milestone. Do I really have to choose between going back to work and celebrating my baby's development and growth, or is the contrast not as severe as it seems?"

- **Black-and-white:** "I was late to work today because I wanted to spend some extra time making food for the baby and forgot about an important morning meeting. I'm going to get fired."

Flexible: "Yes, I messed up this morning. But I've missed a meeting before. All I have to do is send out an email with an explanation and an apology, and not let it happen again, and people will forgive and maybe even forget. I wasn't a perfect employee before, and I don't have to be so hard on myself. In my office, when you're in trouble they usually call you in to talk rather than just firing you, so if I'm in trouble, I'll know it and will be able to turn things around."

• **Black-and-white:** "My boss doesn't have kids, so she won't get it."

Flexible: "The truth is, my boss and I don't see eye-to-eye on everything. Even if she did have kids, it's unlikely that she would approach work/life balance the same way I do. I need to be clear and communicative with her about my scheduling issues around child care, just as I do with everything else. If I can explain my rationale and how I'm going to get my work done, she tends to be reasonable."

You'll notice that in these examples, the flexible thoughts are longer than the black-and-white ones. That's natural—black-and-white thinking is reductive and binary. Flexible thinking takes more time to figure out and express, which is why it requires intentional practice.

Pumping

If you've been breastfeeding and are returning to work, you'll have to make some decisions about pumping or not. Some mothers say that even if they don't enjoy the physical sensation and logistical demands of pumping, it helps them feel more emotionally connected to their babies, especially in those early days of separation. One of our patients said, "Even when I'm not able to be with him, my breast milk is there in my place."

But even in this age of advocacy for equal rights in the workplace, it can be a challenge to find appropriate accommodations for nursing mothers to pump. While U.S. law requires businesses to provide nursing mothers with breaks and space to pump for up to one year after birth, the reality is often challenging. Women have told us about pumping in bathroom stalls and closets. They've pumped in their offices and had someone enter without knocking. They've received eye rolls upon asking to reschedule a meeting.

If your workplace has not made provisions for pumping, speak to your boss and your human resources representative. Are there other women at your workplace who are pumping? Consider approaching your manager together.

In her book *Work, Pump, Repeat* writer Jessica Shortall suggests being proactive: "The top thing I heard from managers and human resources people is that they want to see women propose a plan for pumping, preferably before the baby is born . . . They want to see an employee who has done her best to figure out what she'll need and how to make it work with her job." Frustratingly, it often falls to mothers to advocate for themselves on this issue.

One of our patients described how unexpectedly fierce she felt about pumping at work: "I was so surprised by what a mama bear I turned into. I became really aggressive, and if I noticed any hesitation or skeptical responses from my coworkers, either in terms of space or in terms of schedule, I was pretty blunt: 'If you want women to succeed here and everywhere, you're just going to have to work around this.'"

Pumping impacts not only how you structure your workday but also your time at home, especially at night. Scheduling a pumping session when you could be sleeping may be gratifying, but it may also feel exhausting. If the costs of pumping—monetary, physical, and psychological—are too high, take some time to reflect on both the positive and negative emotions around pumping. If you're pumping because you think you "should," it may be more about your feelings of guilt than what's necessary for your baby. If you think you're depriving your baby by not giving her breast milk, remember that formula is fine. **We agree with Shortall: "Your worth as a mother is not measured in ounces."**

Mother vs. Other: Working and Child Care

No matter what work situation you choose, you and your partner (regardless of how you organize co-parenting) will need some form of child care. Whether you use day care, a nanny or babysitter, or a family member, your child may spend a lot of her time with one or more caregivers other than you.

Each kind of child care has its pros and cons in terms of economics, logistics, and emotions. We don't recommend any one choice as psychologically healthier than any other. As with any decision related to your child, we recommend that you do your research and trust your instincts about any person you're leaving your child with.

That being said, if considering different caretakers causes you to struggle with catastrophic worries about safety, this concern may be more a reflection of your larger fears than an accurate read of any one specific person as high-risk. Try to remember that, as with airplane crashes, the scary, sensational stories about danger and child care workers are statistically rare.

It's natural to feel anxious about your infant's comfort, routine, and well-being when giving up the control of child care to someone else, even if that person is a beloved relative.

Family Help

You should be as explicit with a family member as you would with a caretaker you hired—even more so if the family member doesn't have recent experience with a baby. It's important to communicate about routines, macro and micro, in terms of feedings, sleep, bathing, dressing, and topics like screen time and basic safety rules. No matter how much you love and trust your family member, you should not

make any assumptions, and we recommend that you err on the side of spelling everything out, even writing down requests and rules, especially in the beginning.

One of our patients shared a story about her own mother, who was a loving, involved grandmother and offered to watch the baby for the afternoon. Our patient told us, "My mom is great with kids, so I assumed that when I dropped my son off at her house so that I could go to an appointment, she would be watching him like a hawk because he was crawling everywhere and my mom's house isn't babyproofed. I couldn't believe it later when I came back from my appointment and realized that she had just been letting him crawl around in her living room right next to this electrical cord. I screamed at her for not being more careful and then felt really bad, but I guess she just forgot what it was like to watch a crawling baby who goes like a magnet to the electrical sockets." While a crisis was averted, our patient realized that she had overlooked questions about safety that she never would have skipped with a stranger.

Sometimes relatives who are trying to be helpful can make things more complicated, which can create more work for you as well as painful conflicts. One of our patients said, "It's hard because my mom passed away, and my dad is involved as a grandfather, but he's just not maternal, so he's not so helpful. When I'm cooking dinner and he's watching the baby, he'll run to me and say, 'She's crying,' rather than just picking her up and taking care of her. So I've learned to not ask him to babysit when I'm really distracted because it's just too frustrating for me. You can't give family members jobs they are not

good at or not interested in—if you do, you will be eternally disappointed."

Some family members may offer to help when you almost wish they wouldn't. Maybe your aunt offers to babysit, but she's a smoker, and you don't want her to smoke in your house. Your sister offers to take your baby for a night while you and your husband go to a wedding, but she puts the baby to bed with a pacifier, and you've been trying to break that habit for your son.

Being clear about your expectations and setting boundaries in these kinds of relationships can be hard but also necessary. We recommend you try to walk the line between holding your authority and respecting your family members. Especially if they are volunteering, you may not be able to control everything they do. Think about what deviations from your parenting style are minor and which are deal breakers. If you're feeling like the differences in approach are intolerable and communication doesn't help, you might want to look into other options. For some families, the price of professional child care is worth the gain of a more professional relationship and routine.

Hiring a Child Care Professional

Even once you decide on professional child care, there are still decisions to be made. Day care can be more affordable than one-on-one babysitting; the group environment with multiple caregivers can provide more social stimulation for your child; and an expanded circle of care can be enriching. Many day care centers provide creative

and educational programming and are well organized about how the day is structured.

For those who can afford it, hiring an individual child care professional, babysitter, or nanny may provide flexibility and convenience. Yet some mothers worry that their baby's attachment to a nanny will interfere with or supplant their baby's attachment to them.

While children can become tremendously attached to loving caregivers, we want to reassure you that, as the mother, you are irreplaceable. Studies have shown that children can love their caregivers and parents at the same time, and that a strong bond to a caretaker only reinforces a baby's healthy attachment to her mother, because she feels loved, safe, and secure regardless of who is home. In other words, children have enough love to go around for multiple caretakers. Studies show that the more love a child gets, from however many caretakers, the better.

If you choose a nanny or daily babysitter, this person may be working inside your home (unless you're bringing the baby to them or have a shared arrangement with another family). This can feel like a more intimate child care relationship. It's important to reflect on whether this type of closeness feels comfortable for you, as your child care professional may become an integrated and central part of your family. **The most successful child care partnership, like any important relationship, is one in which there is good communication and mutual respect.** This requires self-awareness, trust, and openness on your part.

Everyone loses when you can't communicate directly, even

during hard conversations. If your child care worker fears that you might be critical rather than collaborative, she may avoid telling you important details about your child's behavior or her own work schedule, and may be more likely to quit. And if you're afraid to ask the child care worker to do something differently, your child may not get the care you want her to have, and miscommunications may begin to add up. If you're avoiding these hard conversations, you need to figure out what your fear of more direct communcation is *really* about.

How to Maintain a Healthy Relationship with Your Child's Caregiver

- **Assess your baggage:** Talk to your partner, friends, or anyone else you trust about any preexisting issues you may be stressed about. Are you angry at your job for unaccommodating policies? Resentful that your spouse doesn't carry more of your family's financial burden? If you can, try to address these problems at their source (talk to your boss about your schedule, talk to your partner about the family income and budget, talk to your parents about what your childhood was like; or find a friend or therapist to talk to about any of the above). Reflecting on what you're really upset about may help prevent you from projecting these feelings on to the caregiver.

- **Be fair:** You and the child's caregiver should both be clear about your expectations. Follow a written contract that is respectful to both parties. Look to groups like the National Domestic Workers Alliance for ethical employer guidelines (see **Resources**). The more mutual trust and respect you and the caregiver share, the better you will be able to work together to help your child.

- **Keep communication direct and open:** Create an environment in which your child's caregivers feel comfortable talking to you. You should feel comfortable discussing your own requests, including asking them to change any approaches to child care that aren't consistent with your parenting style. And they should be comfortable coming to you with questions and concerns as well, both about your child as well as the logistics of their job.

- **Work together to put the children first:** Make your caregivers your partners. Ask them to send you photos or videos of your child throughout the day. Tell them when you're thinking about trying new feeding, sleeping, or behavioral approaches, and educate them about your philosophy so they can be inspired to get on board. If you notice they're resisting your requests, ask them about it. You may learn something from their parenting approach that you hadn't considered, or something about their culture or family upbringing that can sensitize you to their perspective and help you respectfully explain your different style. You can do this whether you have a single caregiver, multiple babysitters, or use day care. We recognize that this isn't always easy, but the work is always worth it.

Friendship, Competition, and Unsolicited Advice

When you become a mother, some of your focus inevitably shifts from the adults in your life to your child. When you try to reengage with your social life, the logistics of daily life with a baby can be unpredictable, and even with all the best intentions, you may see less of your friends.

If you have friends with babies, you may find that you spend more time with them than other friends, simply because you're at the same stage of life and have the same concerns. For some mothers, other parents they meet during these early years become lifelong friends, sharing in parenting pleasures and concerns, supporting each other, and simply providing adult stimulation during hours sitting together on a play mat or at the playground.

Because new motherhood can be a reclusive and overwhelming time, you may not have time, energy, interest, or ability to coordinate and connect with friends who do not have children or whose children are at a different life stage. Some of your friends will be more patient and understanding than others. A friend's avoidance may be due to a lack of interest in babies or your new routine. Friends who may be struggling with older children, infertility, or longing for children may avoid you because of their own emotional challenges.

While it's understandable to feel hurt, we encourage you to try waiting it out with these friends. They may need some time to see that you're still you, even if the logistics of how you hang out have changed. If you are able and interested in persevering, keep inviting them and give them a chance to regroup.

Sometimes, however, a friendship cannot be repaired; the disagreements and physical or emotional distance may be too great. If that happens, let yourself grieve the loss of someone who was important to you. You may also find that you gravitate toward different people in this phase of life, at least for a few years. As your identity expands and changes, your friendships will continue to evolve with you.

One of our patients found that her interest in talking to other parents fluctuated during certain phases with her baby: "When things were going well, I loved swapping tips with other mothers. But as soon as we started sleep training, I couldn't handle hearing anyone's advice. My good friend had sleep-trained her baby in just three nights, but my daughter was so much more difficult. Suddenly, all I wanted when I saw my friend was to talk about anything *other than* our babies. I felt really lucky that I could just say to her: 'Things are really rough right now, I just need to talk about something else!'"

Competition is a common social tension that we hear about

from new mothers. As with any other time in life, some people, consciously or not, may find a way to turn the conversation to prove that they have it the best, or even the worst. Maybe you're commiserating about how tired you are, and your friend one-ups you with stories about how her sleep deprivation is being compounded by her demanding (and impressive) accomplishments at work or full social calendar.

Competitive friends are usually not trying to put you down but, rather, trying to make themselves feel better. **When it comes to parenting, there are very few "right" answers, and that makes everyone feel insecure about their decisions.** It's easy to pass judgment on others if you're trying to defend your own choice to yourself, or are trying to downplay your own fears. One of our patients said, "I'm a perfectionist, so it took me a really long time to believe there wasn't actually a best way to deal with any particular issue with the baby, or all babies. It was really freeing when I realized that whatever you do, some things will go well, some things will be a mess, but if you're basically able to keep your eyes open and make sure things are safe, the baby will always be fine."

Maybe you've been having issues with breastfeeding for weeks, and you've tried every intervention, and your friend tells you to "just relax" in a dismissive way. Our patients tell us that "just relax" is one of the most unhelpful things you can hear as a nervous new mom. Even if you know that someone is just trying to help you feel at ease, it's frustrating and invalidating when you *want* to be able to relax but simply feel wound up. Furthermore, when someone says "just relax," it can feel like a high-pressure command that actually interferes with your ability to let go, like telling someone with insomnia to "just go to sleep." If a well-intentioned friend is telling you to "just relax" in response to your venting about a parenting problem, you can ask him to just listen, or you can explain how counterproductive that advice really is.

We suggest you build a team, real and virtual, of accredited experts and trusted friends and family you can go to for information, advice, and the occasional reality check. Choose the people who not only have the best advice but also communicate in a way that makes you feel supported. Your aunt may be a pediatric nurse, but if she goes to the worst-case scenario, making you feel panicked when you call about your baby's runny nose, she may not be the best person to call if your baby falls and bumps her head.

We think it's important that mothers try to catch themselves before they criticize each other. One of our patients said, "Before I had a baby, I was so judgmental of parents I saw out in the world. I hated when people brought babies to restaurants—they'd just start crying or make a mess, and I would think that the parents clearly didn't know what they were doing and that I would never let my child be so out of control. But now that I'm a mother, I know every parent is just trying to do their best. And if anyone is judging me, I think, *Who cares? They don't know my life or my baby. Why does a stranger's opinion matter to me?*"

What unites us as mothers is much stronger than differences of opinion or parenting styles: Every mother wants what's best for her child, even if how she gets there doesn't always look the same. If women are going to continue to advance in equality, none of us can afford to waste our energy on "mommy wars."

If you don't have many friends with babies around the same age as yours, or you're looking for more support or connection, the internet has much to offer. There are parenting message boards, blogs, Facebook groups, listservs, and more. Especially when it's hard to leave the house, these groups can create supportive communities and offer helpful resources. But so many moms sharing their stories in one place can also be overwhelming. Since no baby is like another, we encourage you to be cautious about online advice. Just because other moms had success with a certain approach doesn't mean it will work for you. It's like trying to find the perfect pair of jeans online: No matter how good they look on someone else, you won't know if they fit until you try them on for size.

Parenting communities on social media can be fun, distracting, and supportive. But social media can also bring out extremes: people who are interested in sharing their horror stories, and those who are know-it-alls or "bliss-mythers," moms who refuse to acknowledge anything negative about their parenting experience. Social media can trigger low self-esteem and increase feelings of shame. If you find that you're feeling low after spending time online, take a day or two off and see if it helps you feel better. You won't be missing much, and your friends know where to find you.

Returning to Your Sex Life

Whatever your sexual dynamic was before you had the baby—how often you had sex, who initiated it, what you enjoyed or didn't—may have changed since you've had a baby. Your partner may be eager to reconnect intimately, but you may feel differently. Your doctor may clear you for sexual activity at your six-week checkup, though at that point, you may feel far from healed from childbirth and not yet ready for sex.

Your postpartum body may feel less like a wonderland and more like a battle zone. If you've delivered vaginally, you may worry that you've been "stretched out," or you may feel dry. A C-section scar may be healed but still visible and tender. If you're nursing, you may experience your breasts as a sexual turnoff if they're leaking or simply because you've been relating to them in such a nonerotic way. Emotionally and physically, you probably still don't feel like yourself, so it may be challenging to feel "hot" the way you use to. If you've been caring for the baby all day—especially if you're nursing—you can feel like you've been touched to death, and the last thing you want is someone coming at you, putting something where you don't want it put right now. Or you may be in the mood for sex but too exhausted to do anything about it by the time the baby's asleep.

There may be evolutionary roots for a diminished interest in sex during the first year postpartum: You're focusing your energy on caring for your baby, and that leaves less for other pursuits, especially pursuits that, biologically, could produce another baby for you to take care of. There's also a hormonal explanation for a lack of interest in sex, even after the medically approved waiting period. One of our patients told us what she craved was the rush that being skin-to-skin with her baby gave her, not her partner. All the cuddling and holding your baby (and breastfeeding, if you're doing that) releases oxytocin in your brain. Oxytocin is the same bonding hormone that is released during orgasm. When you get it from one source, you may not want it from another.

But if your partner isn't getting the benefit of those same oxytocin surges, he may be longing for more intimacy with you. While he may not be aware of feeling rejected or envious of the baby, he may express his dissatisfaction in subtle ways: withdrawing to his phone or other devices, spending more time away from home with friends or at work, or even "eating his feelings," which might explain why many partners gain weight in new parenthood.

Your partner's sexual advances are more than just a sign of neediness for your body and love. They're also a way for him to say that he still values you as a romantic partner. It's healthy to try to hold on to your identities as lovers in addition to being partners and parents. If sex is an important way you normally bond, but you don't want it yet, try to continue some forms of physical contact, for example: holding hands and kissing each other good night. Your sexual connection isn't only about sex—it's also about closeness and communication. And it's one of the foundations of your relationship, not as parents, but as people who love each other.

How to Be Creative About Sex in the Postpartum

- **Communication is foreplay.** Before you have sex for the first time after childbirth, speak honestly with your partner about how you're feeling, physically and emotionally—even or especially if you're not sure how you're feeling. Your partner may feel the same way. Talk about what you want and what acts or positions you may not be ready for yet. Remember you have many options beside penetration. Let him know what you need to feel comfortable, and don't be surprised if things are awkward at first. With patience, love, and a sense of humor, you will figure it out.

- **Cuddling counts.** Just as skin-to-skin is healthy for your body with your baby, consider taking a shower together or spooning your partner in bed with your clothes off, and enjoying reconnecting by stroking her hair or massaging her back even if you're not ready for genital touching. Maybe you'll enjoy a backrub not as a prelude to sex but just to feel good. Try not to be goal-oriented about sex or achieving orgasm. So much about getting your sex life back is simply about reconnecting with intimacy and touch.

- **It's okay to be a giver.** If you don't want to be sexually stimulated, ask your partner if you can pleasure her body without reciprocation. If the imbalance makes her feel uncomfortable, ask for something else you may want, like a foot rub.

- **Feel yourself first.** If you're worried about pain from intercourse, experiment first with your own fingers or a vibrator to see what it feels like. Being in control during masturbation may help you relax as you get to know your post-pregnancy body and sexual responsiveness.

- **Don't forget to turn yourself on.** Maybe you need to make yourself feel sexy in order to feel sexual—if you used to groom your body hair or wear lingerie before pregnancy, see if doing that gets you in the mood, even if it feels like the last thing you have time for. Treat yourself to some new underwear to complement your current shape. Wear a bra that makes you feel attractive if you're feeling self-conscious about your changed breasts or leaking. Speaking of which, have some towels on standby, and try to laugh rather than cry over spilled milk.

- **Use lube.** Vaginal dryness is common in the postpartum period. Speak to your doctor if you have any specific questions about your healing and how to make sex feel more comfortable.

- **Take care of the baby first.** Do your best to feed, change, and put the baby to sleep with a full tummy so she doesn't wake you up and you aren't distracted by thoughts about her needs.

A baby's schedule, or lack of it, can put a damper on sex. You might finally feel like having sex, but it's at the same time the baby wants to nurse. If your baby is sleeping in the same room, you may worry that you are traumatizing her if she wakes up. While we hear that fear a lot, try not to worry too much: Even if she sees what you and your partner were doing, an infant won't understand what's happening.

We've found that in the first year of parenthood, and often for some time beyond, a disparity of desire between mothers and their partners is common. But as frequent as it is, lack of sex can be a major factor in creating distance in a couple. **You may not realize how important your sexual connection is to your communication until it goes away.** It's not just about the physical intimacy; often during "pillow talk," couples reveal and resolve minor conflicts that could become major irritants if they weren't addressed.

One of our patients said, "After our baby was born, my husband was so irritable. I thought it was sleep deprivation, but even getting more sleep didn't help. Once we got our sex life back—in some form—a lot of that tension melted away. He was so much more patient with me, and was even more engaged with the baby. Being sexually connected again made him feel like he and I were a team—and that the baby wasn't an impediment to our relationship."

For some couples, a sexual time-out isn't devastating. They see it as a phase that they will get through. But don't assume your partner will intuit why you're not interested; it's better to talk about what's going on to avoid hurt feelings and becoming alienated from each other.

Many of our patients have shared a fear that if they stopped having sex, it would push their partner away, even toward infidelity. In a mature relationship, your partner would share his feelings before acting out. But the reality is that sometimes a partner may seek physical comfort elsewhere if he experiences a lack of sex as your lack of desire for *him*.

One of our patients came from a family with a history of infidelity and was worried that her disinterest in sex would drive her husband to cheat. She told us, "I was able to talk to my husband about it, and he was really reassuring and explained that he would just tell me if he was losing his mind with sexual frustration—he would never go behind my back and cheat. So sometimes he would tell me or just try to initiate. I wasn't always interested initially, but we figured out things to do so that I was comfortable." When this patient confessed her situation to a friend, it turned out the friend had gone through the same thing: "She told me that she and her husband called it 'outercourse.' It wasn't what we'd done before, but it was enough to keep us bonded until things went back to normal."

While you may choose to have sex with your partner even if you're not feeling turned on, guilt or coercion is not part of a healthy relationship. No one should have sex when he or she doesn't want to. If you've experienced sexual trauma, be especially protective of yourself in this way. If having sex is uncomfortable physically or emotionally, be direct and tell your partner. And if you're really confused about a change in your sex drive, this is a good question to bring to your practitioner. There may be a medical reason and intervention that can be helpful.

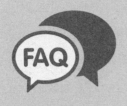

Your personal circumstances will affect the questions that come up for you during your baby's first year. Here are a few that we've been asked most often:

When should I start thinking about having another baby?

It's rare that we hear mothers talk about having another child in the first months after a baby is born. At three months, you may be at your most sleep-deprived and actively wishing to never go through this again. But at twelve months, your baby is bigger and more independent; your body has recovered (more or less); and your period has likely returned. Parenting may start to be more fun, and the toddler your baby will be soon is on the horizon.

You may be concerned about your age and fertility; you may know it took a long time to get pregnant the first time and want to give yourself plenty of time. Or you might be wanting a large family, inspired by your own closeness with your many siblings. Whatever your motivation, you may still want to consider waiting until your baby has his first birthday before you start trying to get pregnant again.

If you're concerned about your fertility, speak with your obstetrician. Most doctors will tell you not to rush into another pregnancy. There are several compelling reasons for this: Your hormones and cycle may be unpredictable if you're breastfeeding; you may be physically recovering from your last pregnancy; and the exhaustion involved in caring for an infant could take a toll on your sex life and stress levels. If you feel like your biological clock is pressed for time but you're not ready to plan your next pregnancy, you can meet with a fertility doctor to discuss your options. If you went through fertility treatments for your previous pregnancy, you want to be completely recovered from the birth and in good health before you undertake them again.

From a psychological standpoint, you've been pretty busy caring for an infant and coping with the significant changes of matrescence. **Give yourself the opportunity to honor this process before you have to do it all over again.** And remember how little control you have over *when* you become pregnant. It could take months, or it could occur the first time you try. One of our patients decided to start trying for a second child when her first was just six months old: "It took us a year to get pregnant the first time, so we figured we might as well get started." Long story short, her two children are a mere fifteen months apart.

Or you may decide that one child is the right number for you. If that's the decision you and your partner agree on, you don't have justify or explain it to anyone else.

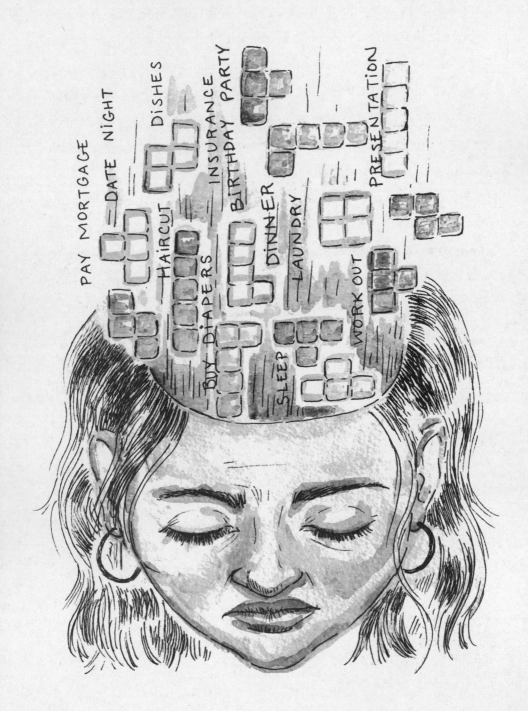

Conclusion: Happy Birthday to YOU!

With your baby's first birthday comes a bittersweet ending to babyhood. He will never be so physically dependent on you again. This may bring a sigh of relief but also some sadness, as you pack up the tiniest onesies that he'll never wear again. In addition to feeling sentimental, we hope you also feel joy. And as you celebrate his first year, we encourage you to celebrate yourself, too.

You've made it through pregnancy and the first year of your baby's life and your matrescence! You've been through some of the most dramatic physical, hormonal, and emotional changes a person can go through, and you've emerged with a new family and a new identity. You've nurtured another human being and been transformed by the process. Even if you've struggled this year, you've changed and grown in profound ways, acquiring new skills and a new level of resilience.

There may be moments when you wish you had your old life back. But the paradox of letting go means there's now space for new experiences. You'll spend a lot of time sitting on the floor playing with blocks, but motherhood will also expand your world. You'll meet new friends at your child's school, the park, or the playground. You'll enjoy the world through your child's sense of wonder, slowing down to really look at the colors on a bird's feathers and rediscovering old pleasures like jumping in puddles.

We hope you can find a quiet moment to look around at your new life. You don't have to say goodbye to the pre-baby you forever. Introduce her to your new self. Let them hang out a little and get to know each other. Sooner than you think, your child will begin to develop a life of her own. She may need you less, or at least in different ways, and you will have the opportunity to reclaim parts of yourself that you may have put aside, and even create new ones.

We would love to hear from you on your journey. You can find us on social media to continue the conversation.

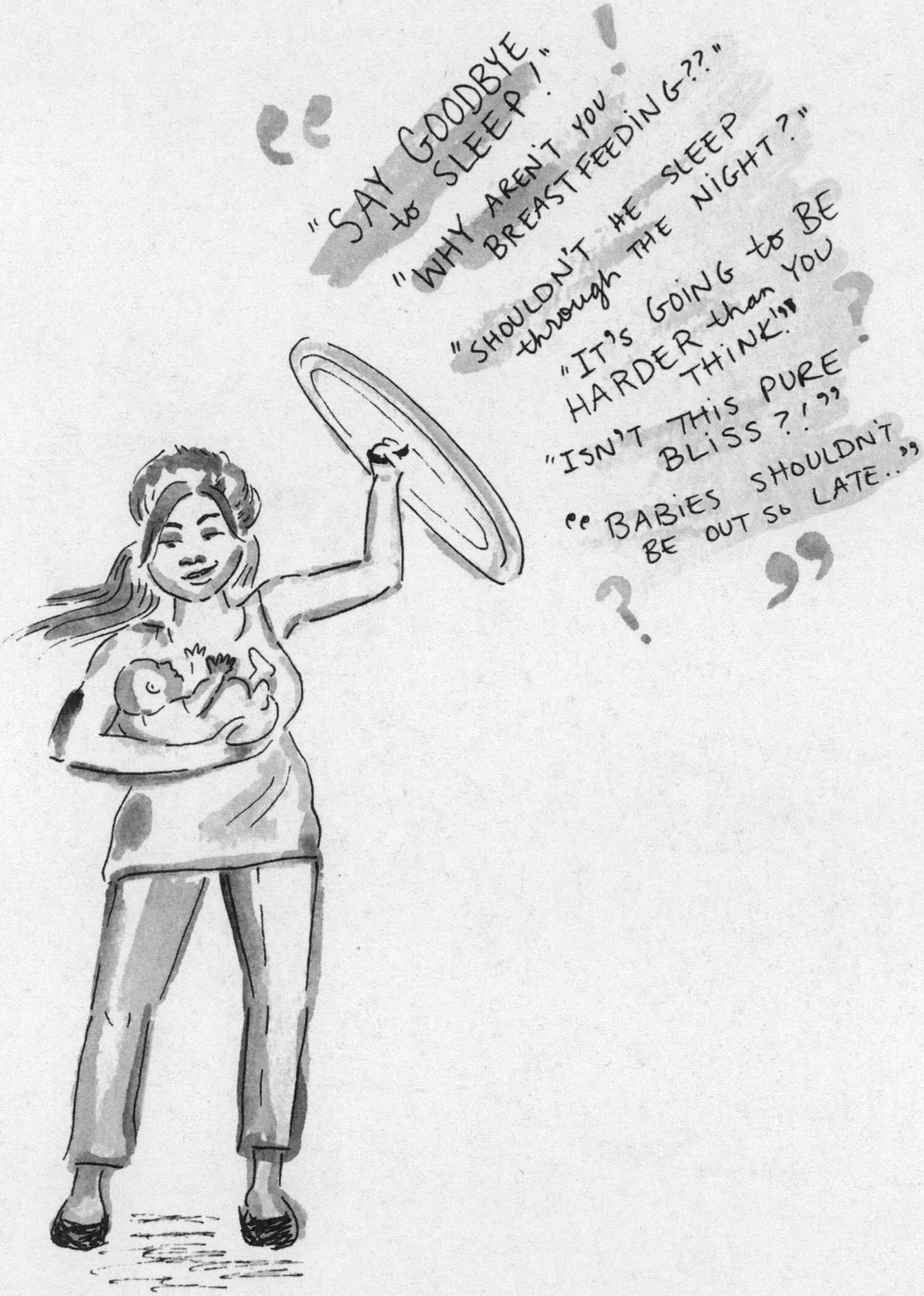
"SAY GOODBYE to SLEEP!"
"WHY AREN'T YOU BREASTFEEDING??"
"SHOULDN'T HE SLEEP through THE NIGHT?"
"IT'S GOING to BE HARDER than YOU THINK!"
"ISN'T THIS PURE BLISS?!"
"BABIES SHOULDN'T BE OUT SO LATE.."

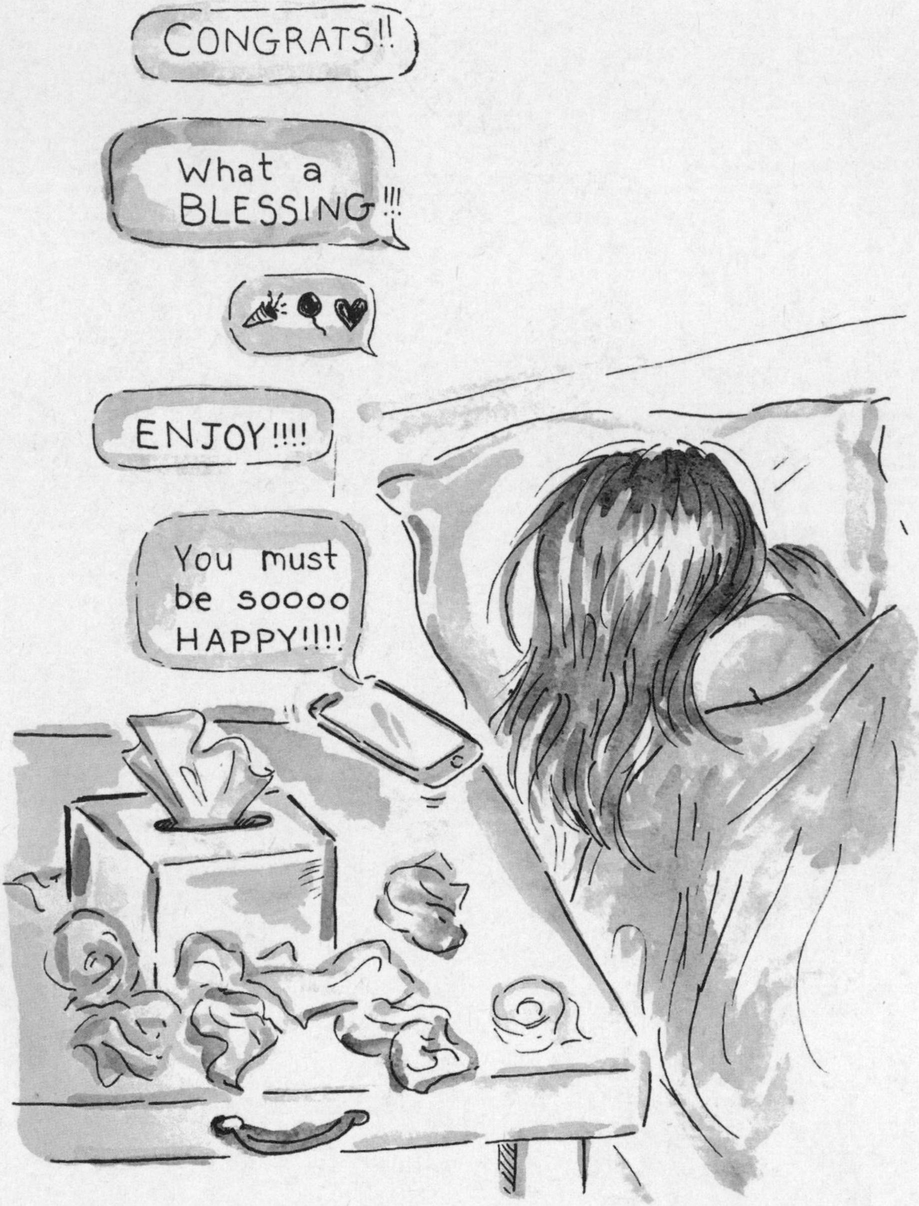
CONGRATS!!
What a BLESSING!!!
ENJOY!!!!
You must be soooo HAPPY!!!!

Appendix

Baby Blues, Postpartum Depression, and Antidepressants During Pregnancy and Breastfeeding

No matter how happy you are about new motherhood, your joy cannot necessarily protect you against clinical depression and anxiety, especially if you are predisposed to these conditions. **However, you don't have to choose between your motherhood and your mental health.** Mothers need proper mental health care during pregnancy and the postpartum period, for their own health and for their baby's, because the wellness of a mother and child are inextricably connected.

Many of our patients have dealt with clinical depression and anxiety for years. They often want to know if the hormonal shifts of pregnancy and postpartum will cast them back into their most difficult times.

Those who have figured out a routine to manage their symptoms prior to motherhood want advice on how to maintain their wellness once the stresses of motherhood arrive. And those who have found stability on an antidepressant or another medication want advice about whether it's safe to continue during pregnancy and breastfeeding.

If you have taken a psychiatric medication in the past or are currently on one, and you are planning a pregnancy or are currently pregnant, we recommend that you set up an appointment with a doctor to discuss your history and options before making any changes on your own. If you're not yet pregnant, you may want to wait to delay your pregnancy (as much as that's possible) until you come up with a plan for how to manage all your health issues, including psychiatric ones.

Some women with a history of mild episodes of depression or anxiety can go off their medications and stay stable when supported by talk therapy and other protective treatments and behaviors. However, studies have shown that stopping your antidepressants before or during pregnancy may result in a relapse of symptoms for up to 65 to 70 percent of women, especially if they aren't being supported by other therapies. For many women with a history of clinical depression or anxiety, research has shown that the combination of talk therapy and medication may work the best to keep symptoms at bay.

Whether you've experienced symptoms of mental illness in the past, are concerned about new symptoms, or want to educate yourself so that you can keep an eye out for symptoms in the future, this chapter is intended to help you feel more prepared.

The "Baby Blues" and the Natural Mood Swings of Matrescence in the Postpartum

Up to 80 percent of women will experience the "baby blues" in the first couple of weeks after childbirth. The baby blues are not mental illness. They are thought to be a natural and temporary reaction to the hormonal shifts that follow childbirth. Many women describe them as a more intense version of PMS. While crying is a symptom, many women with the blues say they feel more emotionally sensitive than sad. Mood swings and irritability are common. The symptoms tend to be worst the first week after delivery and usually go away on their own within two weeks.

Even though they are not dangerous, the baby blues may still be uncomfortable and unsettling. We recommend that you line up support from family, friends, and childbirth professionals like doulas for your own comfort and to help with the baby's care in the first couple of weeks postpartum. But you shouldn't need any professional mental health treatment in order to feel better, because the blues will lift without intervention.

Everyone feels unsteady from time to time—sometimes for an afternoon, sometimes for longer—and new mothers are no exception. You're stressed and spending hours a day with a sometimes screaming baby. Maybe you wish your partner were more domestic, or that your parents lived closer, or that your grandmother were still alive to meet your baby. These feelings come and go in the common course of matrescence.

Simply put, just because you're not happy all the time during pregnancy and new motherhood doesn't necessarily mean that you have symptoms of mental illness.

What Are Clinical Depression and Anxiety?

For most medical conditions that affect the body, the diagnosis is binary: You either have it, or you don't. There are tests that confirm everything from pregnancy to a strep throat. Pee on a stick, get a throat culture, and there's a clear answer, yes or no. But diagnostic tests for illnesses of the mind and brain such as depression and anxiety aren't always as clear-cut. While these are real medical conditions, and there are many diagnostic tools at our disposal, the line between moodiness and a mental health problem can be seen as somewhat subjective, since it is defined by your own experience and the way your emotions are affecting your life.

During matrescence, as in other times of transition, complex feelings, including sadness, will come and go. But sometimes they don't pass. Sometimes your low mood is persistent, inescapable, and seems to have nothing to do with triggers in your daily life. Sometimes you feel sad even while going through experiences that, at any other time, would make you feel happy. It's as if a black cloud is following you everywhere you go. If that dark mood leads to even darker thoughts, a feeling of hopelessness may convince you that there's no use trying to feel better. Sometimes the heaviness of that feeling weighs you down so much that getting through your normal daily routine becomes exhausting or impossible. That's when you may have depression.

Depression is more than just persistent sadness, though that is one of its main symptoms. Rather than feeling dark, depression can feel empty and blank. You may feel "flat," as if the world—and your emotional life—has gone from color to shades of gray. This is in part because of what happens to the brain during a depressive episode: **It's as if the machine that runs your natural pleasure system is broken.** This flatness can be even more uncomfortable than a feeling of sadness. You may feel unmotivated, disinterested, and disconnected, even from things that you would normally love, like listening to music or eating your favorite ice cream. Sleep may become your only refuge, which is why many people with depression struggle to get out of bed.

Anxiety, a feeling of jittery nervousness, like you're wound up or in danger, often comes along with depression. You may have an ongoing monologue of worries or berating thoughts criticizing you all day long, making it hard to concentrate. Other times, anxiety may be a physical experience, disconnected from conscious worry: tension in your muscles, irritation in your digestion, tightness in your chest, pounding heart, shortness of breath, sweaty restlessness, and an inability to sleep are common. All these symptoms often occur in combination.

Some people have anxiety alone, without depression. You may be a worrier who fears the worst-case outcomes for mundane daily events. Or you may have specific phobias that trigger panic attacks that make you feel short of breath. Sometimes anxiety alone causes you to start feeling depressed—living in that constant state of tension can become so depleting that it may burn out your pleasure system. Worry and sadness are natural in life and during matrescence. But anxiety and depression become a disorder when they interfere with your ability to function and experience any forms of pleasure.

Rx In Our Patients' Words: What Do Depression and Anxiety During Pregnancy and in the Postpartum Period Feel Like?

- **Exhausting Fears of Danger:** "After my son was born, he seemed so fragile. Every time I looked at him, I had a thought of something horrible happening: that there'd be black mold in our air conditioner, that he would develop reflux and lose weight, that if I wasn't on guard, he would stop breathing. When I was giving him a bath, my hands looked so big next to his body—I had these horrible images of him drowning in the water, like nightmares, but I was awake. I couldn't fall asleep because I couldn't turn off these worries. Eventually I stopped wanting to make plans, leave the house, or even get dressed because I was so drained; everything just felt like too much and like there was too much risk for danger everywhere."

- **Depleting Self-Criticism:** "I had some bleeding early on in my pregnancy. I felt guilty that working out is what caused the problem, even though my doctor said that it wasn't anything I did wrong. Even after my doctor told me it was okay to go back to the gym, I just couldn't feel safe about it. I lost my interest in working out, which is a pretty big deal for me because it's the main way I burn off stress. I couldn't get rid of these guilty thoughts that I was already a selfish mom because I hadn't rested more in the beginning, and that my baby deserved better."

- **Loss of Pleasure, Trouble Concentrating, Social Isolation:** "Breastfeeding was working, I was physically healing, and my partner was a total trooper. But all I could think about was *when's the next diaper change, when's the next feeding.* Nothing was fun or enjoyable. Life became a running to-do list, and I was just going through the motions. I felt pretty worthless—just ugly and fat and irritable. I wasn't even able to concentrate when I was watching TV; all I wanted to do was stay in bed and hide under the covers and be alone."

- **Irritability, Hopelessness, and Tears:** "I thought I just had the baby blues, but my son was already two months old, and I was still always on edge, snapping at my boyfriend for no real reason. I broke down crying with my mom one day because I completely lost hope; I even thought that the baby might be better off without me. She told me that she'd felt the same way after I was born. She said, 'It doesn't have to be as hard as it was for me,' and came with me to my doctor to talk about how I was feeling."

Perinatal Mood and Anxiety Disorders

We have heard the terms "postpartum depression," "postpartum anxiety," "PPD," and "postpartum" used interchangeably to cover a wide range of conditions. Mental health professionals are moving toward a more inclusive term: perinatal mood and anxiety disorders (PMADs). "Perinatal" means "around pregnancy," and PMADs include postpartum depression, anxiety, post-traumatic stress disorder, obsessive-compulsive disorder, bipolar disorder, psychosis, and other psychiatric conditions, all of which can occur separately or in combination during and after pregnancy.

We are going to focus on the most common perinatal mental illnesses that we treat: perinatal anxiety and depression. If you'd like to learn more about the other PMADs, please see our **Resources.**

Postpartum depression and postpartum anxiety typically begin in the first two to three months postpartum, but many of the women who suffer from these conditions actually begin to experience symptoms *during* pregnancy. This is why we prefer the term "perinatal" to "postpartum."

Depressive Disorder

Major depressive disorder is a disease that may include some or all of the following symptoms during pregnancy or the postpartum period. When these symptoms occur in a cluster and last for two weeks or more, that's an indication that you should go speak to a professional about diagnosis and treatment. The following are the most common symptoms:

- Depressed, sad, anxious, or "empty" mood
- Tearfulness
- Loss of interest in usual activities
- Feelings of guilt
- Feelings of worthlessness or helplessness
- Fatigue
- Irritability
- Feeling slowed down or restless
- Sleep disturbance
- Change in appetite
- Poor concentration
- Suicidal thoughts

Anxiety Disorders

Unlike major depressive disorder, which refers to one condition, there are many different conditions that fall under the umbrella term "anxiety disorders." Here are some common features:

Worries that cannot easily be soothed and border on irrational. They may be persistent and relate to health and safety, especially the baby's. For example, you may be worried about whether the baby is getting enough milk from breastfeeding even if your pediatrician has already assured you that the amount and the baby's growth and health are healthy.

Obsessional thoughts describe when a worrisome idea or image sticks in your head and repeats over and over in a loop. If there is a certain behavior or thought you find yourself repeating to try to calm that worry (and the behavior is excessive and doesn't realistically put the worry to rest), we call that a compulsion. When this cycle takes up significant time and energy, it is thought of as a disorder, and may be diagnosed as **Obsessive-Compulsive Disorder.** Our patients tell us that a common obsession is repeated worrying about the baby's breathing at night; a common associated compulsion is staying up all night to watch or count the baby's breaths. Obsessive worries about germs may lead to compulsive cleaning or googling about illness. These thoughts can intrude upon daily life and feel disturbing.

Some mothers with these types of worries may fear being alone with their baby, or they may be **hypervigilant or on guard in a way that interferes with their daily enjoyment and routine.** Those suffering from an obsessive-compulsive cycle cannot stop checking their baby at night, even if the pediatrician has already discouraged them from doing this, and even if they would rather sleep than watch the baby all night. However, they find themselves pulled into this repeated uncomfortable behavior and unable to break the cycle.

Many women with postpartum anxiety disorders are troubled by **fears of harm or violence happening to the baby.** Sometimes in these images, women see themselves harming their own baby, like flashes of dropping or drowning the baby. Research has shown that if these thoughts are disturbing to you, they are unlikely to be associated with you acting in a dangerous way. Though you may imagine yourself causing the harm in these scary scenes, if they are upsetting to you, then you can understand them to be more like images where you're playing out your greatest fears rather than anything you would ever act on.

Panic attacks may appear in people whose anxious thoughts take on a physical form, causing uncomfortable feelings in their bodies. Panic attacks often involve intense stress that manifests in physical symptoms like muscle tension, tightness in your chest, shallow and fast breathing, stomach trouble, sweating, and feeling like your heart is quickly pounding. Sometimes panic attacks are so uncomfortable that they lead people to fear they could die.

Post-Traumatic Stress Disorder is another common disorder. Some people experience trauma after witnessing violence, having a near-death experience, losing a loved one, having a birth- or pregnancy-related trauma, or other devastating situations. They may find the event repeating in memories, nightmares, flashbacks, and other stressful emotional and physical sensations. PTSD may also make them feel cut off, on edge, jumpy, irritable, isolated, and generally negative about life, as well as cause trouble sleeping.

When and How to Seek Professional Help

Not all doctors screen for PMADS, though we think they should. Your doctor may be more focused on taking care of your physical needs, and your child's pediatrician on her health and development. Since symptoms of PMADs such as fatigue and trouble sleeping often overlap with some physical symptoms common in pregnancy and in the postpartum period, even a well-intentioned doctor may not recognize the seriousness of your emotional distress. This is not an excuse, but just underscores the importance of speaking up if you're feeling unwell.

One of our patients told us, "My ob-gyn was really rushed. She would come in and ask me questions while she was doing my exam. I had a hard time thinking straight when I was in the stirrups, and before I knew it, she was leaving the room and telling me everything was going great. I didn't really have any time to talk about how anxious I was feeling. She seemed so confident that I looked fine. I thought I didn't have depression because I trusted that she would have caught it, so I thought it must all be in my head. It wasn't until the next visit, when I could have a calmer conversation with the nurse, before getting undressed, that I was able to explain how miserable I was feeling and I was diagnosed with postpartum depression."

Some women with anxiety, depression, and other conditions keep a poker face around their doctors, either because they're embarassed of the symptoms they are experiencing or they are worried about being shamed. Some providers unknowingly discourage their patients from expressing the true extent of their suffering. This can happen with jokes like "You look better six weeks postpartum than I do six years later!" or the wrong type of clinical minimizing: "Trust me, you'll be fine after a glass of wine and a good night's sleep."

Unlike the transitional adjustments of matrescence, a PMAD won't be cured by a good night's sleep. If you are suffering from or concerned that you may have one of these conditions, try to be as direct as possible in describing how you feel. If you're worried that you might have a PMAD, simply tell your provider in a straightforward way, just like you would say, "My knee hurts, can you tell me what's going on?" You can say, "I'm not feeling well emotionally, I need you to help me figure how to feel better." If you find doctors' offices intimidating, write your question down on a piece of paper or as a note on your phone so you can reference it in the exam room, or bring your partner or a friend to the appointment.

Thankfully, practitioners are becoming more educated about PMADs; hopefully, yours will ask during your perinatal visits how you are feeling emotionally. But if it doesn't come up for any reason, or if you begin to feel unwell before or after that appointment, know that you can call any doctor you trust to discuss.

Often, your doctor (likely a primary care or family medicine practitioner or ob-gyn) can recommend a mental health professional. Ideally, you want to speak to someone who has experience working with reproductive mental health issues and PMADs—she'll understand the complicated relationship between mental health and the radical changes you're experiencing in your body, hormones, and your life. But any medical and mental health professional should be able to help clarify your diagnosis and come up with a plan for treatment, or at least point you in the direction of a specialist. **If you can't find someone locally, contact Postpartum Support International (see Resources), an organization that has a help hotline and connects women to mental health providers all over the world.**

Many women have told us that they started to feel more in control after simply setting up their first mental health appointment, because they knew they were no longer alone. Knowing that you have a private, nonjudgmental person on your side, someone who has seen this situation before and has a plan to help you feel better, can be immediately comforting and help restore your hope. Fortunately, the treatments for PMAD are highly effective, and once people get the proper help, many start feeling better within a few weeks.

What to Expect When You Meet with a Mental Health Professional

If you've never seen a mental health practitioner before, it's hard to know exactly what to expect. Mental health care takes many forms. Whether you want coaching, guided exercises, a medication expert, or just someone who will listen, you can find a good fit.

In your first meeting, your therapist may ask a lot of questions—this is, in part, to help her make a diagnosis in the same way that a medical doctor would listen to your breathing with a stethoscope. She may ask you to describe when you started to feel unwell, specifically how your functioning and daily life have changed, and if you've ever felt this way before. She may ask you to tell her about the days that have been the hardest, and if there's anything that has worked to bring you some relief. She may ask you about your family history, and significant events in your past, in addition to your general health history.

If there's anything that feels important but doesn't come up in the conversation, or a secret you've been keeping that you're not sure is safe to share with anyone, do your best to speak up. It can feel scary to tell a stranger your most private, intimate thoughts, but remember that this is what mental health professionals are trained for. They are also required to keep everything you tell them private—even from your spouse. The only exceptions to this rule are if they are concerned about your safety or your risk of hurting someone else.

A Primer on Different Types of Therapists

There are many different types of mental health professionals. Most use talk therapy to treat PMADs, either one-on-one or in a group setting. Only a medical doctor (MD/DO) or a nurse practitioner (NP) can prescribe medication. Here is how to help you understand the different categories of mental health providers:

Therapists (includes: social worker, psychologist, psychotherapist, counselor): These talk therapists are trained in diagnosing and treating a range of emotional problems and conditions. They may focus on your family dynamics and how other aspects of your social life, such as relationships and financial issues, may be factoring in to your stress. They may work on their own or develop treatment plans with medical doctors and other health care professionals who can prescribe medication alongside their treatment. Therapists may have a PhD in a field like psychology, or a master's degree in counseling or social work. Some therapists have special expertise in women's mental health (infertility, postpartum depression, pregnancy loss, etc.). Some therapists are trained in specific types of behavioral therapies or even body work. As with any provider, feel free to ask about her professional background, training, and clinical philosophy as part of your consideration in assessing your comfort.

Nurse practitioner: A registered nurse who has additional training and responsibilities, such as examining patients, diagnosing illnesses, and providing treatment, including psychotherapy and prescribing medication. Some specialize in psychiatric therapy and medications.

Psychiatrist: A medical doctor who diagnoses and treats mental illness. Psychiatrists often use a combination of talk therapy and medication. Some only prescribe medications and partner with therapists who provide counseling.

Reproductive psychiatrist (Like us!): Sometimes called perinatal psychiatrists or consultation liaison psychiatrists, these are medical doctors who are trained in mental health conditions that are associated with the postpartum period (as well as the menstrual cycle), and how to safely treat them.

Women, Pregnancy, and Psychiatric Medication: A Complicated History

Psychiatric medications offer people with symptoms of mental illness relief from their debilitating symptoms. These medications can make lives better—and have undoubtedly saved lives. And yet, historically, the question in the medical community has not been *how* to treat psychiatric illness during pregnancy, but *whether* to treat it at all.

For years, most doctors, including psychiatrists, were reluctant to give pregnant women medication for psychological conditions due to fear of harming the baby. Even today, this reluctance stands, largely because no psychiatric medications are officially Food and Drug Administration (FDA) approved for use during pregnancy and breastfeeding.

Prior to the early 1990s, the medication research trials that determine FDA drug safety ratings largely did not include among their subjects women of reproductive age. This was out of concern that they could become pregnant during the study, or that their hormonal fluctuations could skew the data. The restriction of these women from medical trials meant that there was no way to test the safety of medications for pregnant women. Concerns about medication safety were further heightened by the dangers of thalidomide, a drug used in the 1950s in Europe to treat morning sickness, which resulted in severe birth defects.

The appropriate goal of preventing future tragedies had the unfortunate consequence of limiting medical research on female patients, pregnant and not. Organizing research around male subject pools prevented the study of psychiatric and physical conditions specific to women. Furthermore, it limited the study of how medical conditions might manifest differently in women's bodies (we now know that women's heart attack symptoms, for example, may present differently than men's).

In the early 1990s, legislation finally required the inclusion of more women into clinical trials in the United States, but research on pregnant women was and is still constrained. We still don't have an exact answer to the question "Is this medication safe to take during pregnancy or while I'm nursing?" because research on medication use in pregnant and breastfeeding women continues to be limited. The "gold standard" in medical research trials that the FDA uses to approve drugs (randomized, double-blind, placebo-controlled clinical trials) require large numbers of people to be studied under a controlled and scientifically objective format. This type of research generally isn't conducted on pregnant and nursing women (which may be one of the reasons why the internet is full of terrifying misinformation). This means that we are often lacking in gold-standard research on conditions that effect pregnant women.

However, just because we don't have FDA-approved psychiatric drugs for pregnancy doesn't mean that we don't have any data on the safety of medications during pregnancy (and breastfeeding).

The vast majority of the safety data we have on medical and psychiatric medications during pregnancy is from retrospective-type studies, in which researchers find women who had decided on their own to take medication, and look back to see if any problems resulted for their babies. This research technique is not considered gold standard because it relies on patients' memories (which are not objective), and there is no way to control all the outside factors that may affect health outcomes, like family history or other factors that affect wellness, like catching the flu. But that doesn't mean these studies are not valuable.

By now we have data aggregated from thousands, if not hundreds of thousands of women who have taken antidepressants during pregnancy, and much of this data comes from other countries where pharmacy and patient health information is widely available for researchers to use. In fact, we may now have more data about the safety of antidepressants than we have about most other categories of medication during pregnancy. The data tells us that, like all medical medications, some psychiatric medications carry more risk for a developing fetus than others. The research also shows that there are only a few psychiatric medications that doctors absolutely avoid during pregnancy, because only these few have been clearly associated with birth defects.

Doctors accept that treating life-threatening medical conditions like high blood pressure or diabetes may involve exposing babies to the risk of unknown medication side effects, often because the diseases themselves would create an unhealthy environment for both the mother and the baby.

Treating psychiatric disorders, however, is still sometimes seen as less medically necessary. For years, women were instructed to "tough out" their emotional symptoms. **Today, science has shown that many psychiatric conditions can also be unhealthy for mother _and_ baby if left untreated during pregnancy and in the postpartum period.** Even though the data is not perfect, for many women, the health benefits of taking diabetes medicine, blood pressure medicine, and antidepressants during pregnancy and in the postpartum period outweigh the hypothetical or even known risks that may be associated with our limited research.

Women with untreated depression are more likely to self-medicate with alcohol and cigarettes, which they might not use otherwise if they weren't so desperate for relief. Some theories suggest that untreated depression and anxiety raise a mother's stress hormones, which may lead to physiological changes that may impact the developing fetus. Studies have also shown that pregnant women with untreated depression may be at a higher risk to go into preterm labor or have a baby with low birth weight.

Whether through talk therapy or medication, it's important to treat depression, anxiety, and other mental illnesses during pregnancy and in the postpartum period. Research and our experience have shown that these treatments are effective, and that when a mom is healthy, it's not only better for her, it's best for her baby, too.

Taking Medication During Pregnancy and Postpartum

If you've been treated for a psychiatric condition with medication before or are currently taking one, we recommend that you set up a meeting with your doctor, ideally before you become pregnant or as soon as you find out that you are. In this meeting, you should discuss: What are the ways that this medication has helped you in the past? Do you remember the last time you were off medication? What did it feel like?

If psychiatric medication has been central to your wellness and you've seen the problematic outcomes of trying to go off medication in the past, then you should discuss any specific risks that research has found to be associated with taking that medication during pregnancy and breastfeeding. As reproductive psychiatrists, we often say that there may be relative risks in taking any medication during pregnancy, but it may also be risky to stop your treatment of depression and anxiety, just as it would be to avoid treating high blood pressure during pregnancy.

We won't spell out the specific risks known for any single medication during pregnancy and breastfeeding because there are so many different medications, and the data is constantly being updated; however, our **Resources** section lists some websites that can help educate you about medication use in pregnancy and breastfeeding and direct you to a doctor near you who can help you with this decision.

If you have a psychiatric history, your doctor may focus on the risks and benefits of a medication that has helped you in the past. You may have heard that a particular medication is commonly prescribed for depression during pregnancy. However, the most popular medication may not be the most beneficial one for you. If you haven't taken psychiatric medication before and your doctor is recommending you start one now, your doctor will help you figure out the safest one to try. Doctors usually recommend the lowest effective dose of medication during pregnancy. This does not mean that the lowest dose is always recommended during pregnancy, it just means that you should take the strength of medicine required to keep your symptoms at bay, no more, no less.

Sometimes women become pregnant when they are on a few different psychiatric medications. Ideally, your doctor will help you find a way to treat all your symptoms by maximizing the most effective single medication. Trying to streamline is recommended, because most studies on medication safety look at only one medication at a time. That means that doctors (and the scientific studies they rely on) usually can't tell you much about the risks of taking two or more medications in combination during pregnancy or while you're breastfeeding. So if you're able to effectively manage your symptoms with a single medication, this might be your better choice. For example, many people who take an antidepressant also take a pill for sleep. We often try increasing the dose of a patient's antidepressant to see if it addresses sleep issues so she can be weaned off the sleep aid.

Some women are unsure how much their current psychiatric medication is actually helping them. If you're in this category, you can talk to your doctor about trying to decrease or even wean off your psychiatric medication before getting pregnant, or consider switching to a more effective medication that has a good safety profile for pregnancy.

And if you decide to go off your medication, you shouldn't do it alone—some medications require you be slowly weaned off them to prevent side effects of withdrawal, and this process should take place under the supervision of your doctor.

Ultimately, the choice to continue or stop your medication will be yours (and your partner's, if you choose to include him in this discussion), but an expert opinion can help you understand your options. The bottom line is this: If you have a history of depression or anxiety, or develop a PMAD, you may *need* to take medication during pregnancy or while breastfeeding, because the benefits to you and your baby of treating your condition may outweigh potential relative risks. The health of a mom and her baby are interconnected.

Medication is not a panacea, and it works best in concert with other treatments. When reviewing a patient's risks and benefits of staying on or going off medication during pregnancy and breastfeeding, we always ask: **Are you doing everything you can in terms of your behavior and lifestyle to boost your mood and protect your mental health?**

Some women are able to lower or wean off their medications when they increase their supports (get help around the house, spend more time with nurturing friends or family, start therapy, eat well, get enough sleep and exercise, improve self-care) and reduce stresses (slow down or decrease pressure at work, cut back on personal responsibilities, take the time to relax, avoid people whom you feel like you "should" spend time with but don't want to). Yes, this is easier said than done. Light therapy, yoga, acupuncture, mindfulness, and meditation may also help, but again, may be logistically challenging for some.

If possible, we recommend that patients managing depression and anxiety during pregnancy and in the postpartum try, as much as possible, to put their own wellness first. Can you skip a draining social or family trip? What about telling the committee at your mosque, church, or synagogue that you need a break so you have more downtime to relax on the weekends? Would cutting corners on your weekly errands help? Or asking your boss if you can work from home one day a week? While these approaches may not always be available or realistic, the point is just to treat yourself with TLC whenever possible.

We also ask our patients, whether they are considering medication or not: **Have you tried talk therapy?** While some doctors will prescribe psychiatric medication without talk therapy, we view therapy as a powerful and important complementary tool. It's not a quick fix, often not appropriately covered by insurance, time consuming, and may even be hard to find in your neighborhood. However, for some patients, a helpful talk therapy can treat their symptoms well enough that they are able to safely go off of medications during pregnancy and breastfeeding.

A Primer on Different Types of Therapies

Just as there are different types of mental health professionals, there are different types of talk therapies. Many therapists are trained in more than one of these therapies, and many use a combination of techniques for different situations. A professional may recommend a specific type of therapy that she thinks would be most helpful for you. You can also request a certain type of therapy if you think it would be the most helpful or feel most natural for how you like to communicate or express yourself.

Psychodynamic psychotherapy: Sometimes called insight-oriented therapy, this treatment is related to the concept that unconscious factors influence our emotions and behaviors. The goal is to help you understand how these blind spots prevent you from seeing things clearly and therefore may cause you to repeat problematic experiences. There is often a focus on talking about your past to understand how memories and experiences relate to your current problems. It is designed to help you discover your own answers with your therapist's skilled facilitation.

Psychoanalysis: This is an intensive type of therapy that is a type of psychodynamic treatment. Treatment usually occurs three to five times a week and is often done with the patient lying on a couch. The analyst is a partner who helps the patient become more self-aware by pointing out how patterns of behavior play out in the therapy sessions. This process, called transference, helps the patient to better understand her behavior both with the analyst and with people and patterns in her real life.

Supportive psychotherapy: The therapist uses a more advice-oriented approach to bolster self-esteem and encourage coping strategies. The focus is on feeling and functioning better with specific actions, rather than exploring the root causes of problems.

Interpersonal therapy (IPT): A short-term, structured therapy that helps identify how changes in life can cause stress. The change of identity in new motherhood is a common focus of IPT, but it is also used to help people struggling after other major changes, such as retirement or the death of a loved one. The aim is to help a patient understand that her current distress is a reaction to real-life circumstances and help identify how those life changes have specifically led to stress. There is an emphasis on looking at the quality of relationships and communication skills as a part of feeling better. A therapist may role-play with the patient as a way to work on improving her relationship with herself and others.

Cognitive behavioral therapy (CBT): A short-term and structured therapy focused on how habitual thought patterns can lead to troublesome feelings and behaviors. Specific homework assignments are designed to help patients learn how to look at their unrealistic thoughts more clearly and gain control over them.

Behavioral therapy: This therapy uses positive/negative reinforcement systems to change dysfunctional patterns of behavior and encourage healthier alternatives. It often includes exercises such as relaxation training, stress management, exposure therapy, and biofeedback (using physical signs from your body to get information about and control your mental state), as well as recommendations for behavioral changes like diet and physical exercise to support healing.

Dialectical behavioral therapy (DBT): DBT therapy is often run in groups. It uses techniques similar to those used in CBT, with a focus on learning mindfulness (self-awareness), interpersonal skills, how to control one's emotions, and how to prevent impulsivity and self-harm.

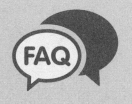

Here are some of the most common questions women ask us about PMADs and the treatment of postpartum depression:

What causes postpartum depression?

Research from the World Health Organization suggests that postpartum depression occurs across cultures and affects 10 to 15 percent of women around the world, with rates highest in developing countries. Centers for Disease Control (CDC) research shows that in the United States, one in nine women may experience postpartum depression. However, some theories suggest that because symptoms may be underreported or unrecognized, the incidences may be even higher.

CDC research shows that women in their childbearing years are roughly twice as likely as men to suffer from depression overall. They're also more likely to have anxiety disorders and PTSD. There are social and psychological theories about how economic inequality, sexual violence, and other cultural patterns may stress women. Other theories suggest that the emotional, physical, and hormonal shifts around pregnancy (and the menstrual cycle) may increase stress in a way that can trigger anxiety and depression.

While scientists don't know the exact cause of PMADs, there are several theories:

After you deliver the baby, your levels of estrogen and progesterone crash. Some scientists believe that the effect of this abrupt hormonal shift on the brain is the cause of baby blues and can contribute to onset of PMADs. However, the story is not that simple. If it were, every woman would go from the baby blues straight into mental illness. **We know that some women are more sensitive to hormonal fluctuations than others.** If you have a history of severe PMS or mood swings on hormonal birth control, you may be more sensitive to hormonal shifts and therefore more predisposed to developing a PMAD.

Some theories suggest that postpartum depression is a form of general depression that occurs during pregnancy and in the postpartum period, perhaps made worse by stress and hormonal shifts, but not a different disease than the type of clinical depression people may experience at other times in life. Sometimes situations of postpartum depression may be a continuation of a depression that has been brewing for some time, even before pregnancy.

There may also be an evolutionary story for PMADs. A burst of healthy alertness encourages a new mother to protect her baby. The nesting urge is an example of this impulse working well. Perinatal anxiety may be that impulse gone awry, or an exaggerated fight-or-flight reaction. These instincts may have been helpful when humans lived on the savanna and had to guard against danger from predators. When these instincts are turned on, even exaggerated, and there's no real danger, it's less productive.

How do I know if I'm at risk for developing postpartum depression?
Before we get into these risk factors, know that they are not a guarantee that you will develop postpartum depression. If you have any

of the risk factors, consider this background an education to help you stay vigilant, put in place support systems, and discuss with your doctor ahead of time.

It may also be helpful to discuss the risk factors for PMADs with your partner, so that she can help you recognize symptoms if they appear. We know that this conversation can be difficult, especially if you have to describe to your partner a history of mental illness struggles that he's never seen. That is another good reason to set up a regular appointment with a confidential professional who may help you feel supported when discussing your past history of mental illness. We encourage our pregnant and postpartum patients to bring their partners to a mental health appointment if they think it would help facilitate their education and communication.

Now for the risk factors: If you've previously suffered from depression or anxiety at another time in life, and/or if you have recently stopped your treatment (including psychiatric medications), you have a higher risk of developing PMADs. **If you've had postpartum depression or anxiety during this pregnancy or a previous pregnancy or postpartum period, the risk for a repeated episode is even higher.**

Like other forms of depression, postpartum depression may have a genetic component. You may be predisposed to develop a PMAD if there is a history of depression in your family, or if other close female relatives have been depressed during pregnancy or the postpartum.

High stress levels can contribute to PMADs. Stressful triggers can include: feeling socially isolated because you're not close to family or friends (or unpartnered), conflict with your partner (including abuse), low self-esteem, financial stress (including stress around child care). Other stressors may factor in, such as prior pregnancy loss, a traumatic birth experience, having your child admitted to the NICU, and struggling with breastfeeding. Sleep deprivation and the adjustments to the many major life changes that occur after a baby is born may also add up as stressors, especially in combination with other risk factors.

Again, we list these risk factors not to worry you but so you can educate yourself, maximize your wellness, and seek preventative help.

When are PMADs an emergency or life-threatening?

If you are having thoughts of suicide, whether it's the urge to commit suicide or just passive thoughts (like wishing that you were not alive or could disappear), you should call your doctor or practitioner right away. If they are not available or do not take you seriously, go to your nearest emergency room or call 911 emergency phone line. If you're feeling unable to ask for professional help, then tell someone you love and trust about how you're feeling and do your best to be honest so that she can understand the severity of your pain and get you the help you need to stay safe.

Another life-threatening subset of PMADs is postpartum psychosis. This disease falls under the umbrella of PMADs but is especially severe and rare, seen in only one or two out of a thousand women after childbirth. Many women who have postpartum psychosis have an underlying psychiatric condition like bipolar disorder.

Symptoms of postpartum psychosis usually come on within the first few days or two weeks after delivery. Symptoms may include dramatic, erratic mood swings, confusion, restlessness, irritability, insomnia, and disorganized or strange behavior. While these symptoms may not sound dangerous, intense displays of emotion may be the external manifestation of the most dangerous aspect of postpartum psychosis: delusional thinking. The delusions of postpartum psychosis may be paranoid or religious, leading the sufferer to think that she or her baby are powerful, dangerous, or in grave danger. Women with postpartum psychosis may hear voices telling them to hurt themselves or their children. And unlike the case of postpartum depression or anxiety, these thoughts of harming themselves or their children may not seem "wrong" in women with postpartum psychosis. In fact, hurting their children may seem like the "right" thing to do as a part of the psychotic delusion.

Postpartum psychosis is a true medical emergency, as women with this condition are at a risk of suicide and infanticide. If there is any question that someone you know may be experiencing postpartum psychosis, you should immediately alert her doctor and family or call 911 or emergency services.

Can fathers and partners get postpartum depression?

Yes. While there has been less research on postpartum depression in fathers, some studies suggest that 4 to 10 percent of fathers may experience depression in the first year after their child's birth. Those with a history of depression may be at higher risk.

Anyone can get depression at any time in life, and just as new parenthood is a stressful time for mothers, the same is true for their partners. Their lives are being disrupted in similar ways: less sleep, less exercise, less sex, less downtime, more responsibility, and more financial pressure. They, too, are facing the excitement and shock of entering a new era of parenthood. We know that stress is one of the most direct triggers for depression and anxiety overall. **Change is stressful for most people, and having a child is a profound change in your partner's life, too.**

Research has not yet clarified if there is a hormonal component to postpartum depression in fathers. Some studies suggest that testosterone levels drop in new dads, and research has shown this pattern in other animal species who parent in pairs, like mice, hamsters, and gerbils. Animal studies show that this decrease in testosterone is correlated with fathers being less aggressive toward their young and more invested in spending time with them, but extrapolations from animal studies to humans aren't perfect. In human fathers, it's unclear if and how hormonal factors may be related to feelings of depression.

As is the case in women, emotional shifts can always be looked at from a biological perspective, and we have a lot to learn about how changes in the body and brain impact our feelings overall for both men and women. Furthermore, it's important to remember that just like mothers, fathers may have a history of depression that preexists parenthood.

There is a growing community of conversation and support for fathers and partners who are experiencing feelings of depression and anxiety in the postpartum period, and a general widening of the conversation about the emotional transition to fatherhood. We also think that many fathers, and families overall, would benefit if paternity/partner leave were more accessible so that partners could have more time at home to bond with their babies, help in their care and in their partner's transition, and have more personal time to rest and adjust.

Resources

We hope these resources will be helpful. However, please note that these web-sites are not under our endorsement and are subject to change. Please also search online for the many wonderful resources where you can connect to other pregnant women and mothers for support virtually and locally.

American College of Obstetrics and Gynecology:

www.acog.org

Breastfeeding/pumping support:

www.womenshealth.gov/breastfeeding/breastfeeding-resources

www.aap.org/en-us/advocacy-and-policy/aap-health-initiatives
/Breastfeeding/Pages/Resources-to-Support-Breastfeeding
-Families.aspx

www.llli.org

Child care supports/advocacy:

www.childcareaware.org

www.domesticworkers.org

mynannycircle.com

Childbirth and postpartum education and healing:

www.cappa.net

www.icea.org

www.dona.org

Financial planning:

www.smartaboutmoney.org

www.singlemomsincome.com

www.benefits.gov

www.thebudgetmom.com

www.ellevest.com

www.usa.gov/benefits

Infertility and pregnancy after assisted reproduction:

www.resolve.org

www.asrm.org

Mental health/psychiatric medications in pregnancy/postpartum:

www.womensmentalhealth.org

www.nimh.nih.gov/health/topics/women-and-mentalhealth
/index.shtml

www.cdc.gov/pregnancy/meds/treatingfortwo

www.motherisk.org

www.mothertobaby.org

www.mindbodypregnancy.com

https://toxnet.nlm.nih.gov/newtoxnet/lactmed.htm

Mental health education and resources:

www.postpartum.net

Phone Help Line English and Spanish:1-800-944-4773. Text
Support: 503-894-9453

National Crisis Text Line: Text HOME to 741741 from anywhere
in the U.S.

National Suicide Prevention Hotline and Website: 1-800-273-
8255

www.suicidepreventionlifeline.org

Mindful meditation and pregnancy/postpartum:

www.mindfulmotherhood.org

www.headspace.com

www.expectful.com

Miscarriage and loss support:

www.compassionatefriends.org

www.nationalshare.org

www.rtzhope.org

www.americanpregnancy.org

Pregnancy and eating disorders:

www.nationaleatingdisorders.org/pregnancy-and-eating
-disorders

Sleep training:

www.healthychildren.org

Support for fathers:

www.postpartumdads.org

www.postpartum.net/family/tips-for-postpartum-dads-and
-partners

www.postpartummen.com

Support for LGBTQ+ parents:

www.gayparentmag.com

www.proudparenting.com

www.gayswithkids.com

Support for parents of twins and multiples:

www.multiplesofamerica.org

Support for parents who adopt or foster babies:

www.adoptioncouncil.org

www.karenfoli.com/#postadoption

Support for single mothers:

www.singlemoms.org

www.singlemothersbychoice.org

https://singlemotherguide.com

Support if you have lost your mother:

hopeedelman.com

Support if your infant has medical needs:

www.marchofdimes.org

www.nationalperinatal.org

Trauma and childbirth:

www.solaceformothers.org

www.ptsdalliance.org

Workers' rights around pregnancy/maternity leave/ breastfeeding:

www.worklifelaw.org

Endnotes

Introduction

Athan, A.M., and H. L. Reel. "Maternal Psychology: Reflections on the 20th Anniversary of Deconstructing Developmental Psychology," *Feminism & Psychology*, 25:3 (2015), 311–25.

Athan, A.M. "Maternal Flourishing: Motherhood as Potential for Positive Growth and Self-development," Lecture Presented at the Women's Mental Health Consortium Quarterly Meeting, October 2016.

Raphael, Dana. *Being Female: Reproduction, Power, and Change.* Chicago: Mouton Publishers, 1975.

Sacks, Alexandra. "The Birth of a Mother," *The New York Times*, May 8, 2017.

———. "A New Way to Think About the Transition to Motherhood," TED Talk, May 31, 2018, https://www.ted.com/talks/alexandra_sacks_a _new_way_to_think_about_the_transition_to_motherhood.

Sacks, Alexandra, Sylvia Fogel, Catherine Monk, Elizabeth Fitelson, Rosemary Balsam. "Matrescence: The Psychological Birth of a Mother from Cognitive and Hormonal Changes to Intergenerational Psychodynamics," panel presented at the American Psychiatric Association Annual Meeting, May 2018.

Stern, Daniel N., Nadia Bruschweiler-Stern, and Alison Freeland. *The Birth of a Mother: How The Motherhood Experience Changes You Forever.* New York: Basic Books, 1998.

Chapter 1: The First Trimester

Brizendine, Louanne. *The Female Brain.* New York: Broadway Books, 2006.

Diaz, Natalie. *What to Do When You're Having Two: The Twins Survival Guide from Pregnancy Through the First Year.* New York: Penguin Books, 2013.

Douglas, Ann. *Trying Again: A Guide to Pregnancy After Miscarriage, Stillbirth, and Infant Loss.* Lanham, MD: Taylor Trade Publishing, 2000.

Johnson, Emma. *The Kickass Single Mom: Be Financially Independent, Discover Your Sexiest Self, and Raise Fabulous, Happy Children.* New York: Penguin Books, 2017.

Oster, Emily. *Expecting Better: Why the Conventional Pregnancy Wisdom Is Wrong—and What You Really Need to Know.* New York: Penguin Books, 2014.

Pepper, Rachel. *The Ultimate Guide to Pregnancy for Lesbians: How to Stay Sane and Care for Yourself from Preconception to Birth.* San Francisco: Cleis Press, 2005.

Raphael-Leff, Joan. *Pregnancy: The Inside Story.* London: Sheldon Press, 1993.

Chapter 2: The Second Trimester

Brown, Sheila Feig. *What Do Mothers Want?: Developmental Perspectives, Clinical Challenges.* Hillsdale, NJ: The Analytic Press, 2005.

Douglas, Ann. *Trying Again: A Guide to Pregnancy After Miscarriage, Stillbirth, and Infant Loss.* Lanham, MD: Taylor Trade Publishing, 2000.

Downey, Allyson. *Here's the Plan: Your Practical, Tactical Guide to Advancing Your Career During Pregnancy and Parenthood.* Berkeley: Seal Press, 2016.

Kohn, Ingrid, and Perry-Lynn Moffitt, with Isabelle A. Wilkins. *A Silent Sorrow: Pregnancy Loss: Guidance and Support for You and Your Family.* New York: Routledge, 2000.

Shahine, Lora. *Not Broken: An Approachable Guide to Miscarriage and Recurrent Pregnancy Loss.* Lora Shahine, 2017.

Weinstein, Ann. *Prenatal Development and Parents' Lived Experiences.* New York: Norton, 2016.

Chapter 3: The Third Trimester

Anderson, Marla V., and M. D. Rutherford. "Evidence of a Nesting Psychology During Human Pregnancy," *Evolution and Human Behavior,* 34:6 (2013), 390–97.

Louden, Jennifer. *The Pregnant Woman's Comfort Book*. San Francisco: Harper Collins, 1995.

Mariotti, Paola, ed. *The Maternal Lineage: Identification, Desire and Transgenerational Issues*. New York: Routledge, 2012.

Maushart, Susan. *The Mask of Motherhood: How Becoming a Mother Changes Everything and Why We Pretend It Doesn't*. The New Press, 1999.

Spinelli, Margaret G. *Interpersonal Psychotherapy for Perinatal Depression: A Guide for Treating Depression During Pregnancy and the Postpartum Period*. Scotts Valley, LA: CreateSpace Independent Publishing Platform, 2017.

Wiegartz, Pamela S., Kevin L. Gyoerkoe, and Laura J. Miller. *The Pregnancy and Postpartum Anxiety Workbook: Practical Skills to Help You Overcome Anxiety, Worry, Panic Attacks, Obsessions, and Compulsions*. Oakland: New Harbinger Publications, 2009.

Chapter 4: Labor and Delivery

The Business of Being Born, directed by Abby Epstein. Barranca Productions, released January 9, 2008.

Campion, Maureen. *Heal Your Birth Story: Releasing the Unexpected*. San Francisco: CreateSpace Independent Publishing Platform, 2015.

Cohen, Erica Chidi. *Nurture: A Modern Guide to Pregnancy, Birth, Early Motherhood—and Trusting Yourself and Your Body*. San Francisco: Chronicle Books, 2017.

Davis, Elizabeth. *Heart and Hands: A Midwife's Guide to Pregnancy and Birth*. New York: Random House, 1981.

Lyon, Erica. *The Big Book of Birth*. New York: Plume, 2007.

Mohrbacher, Nancy, and Kathleen Kendall-Tackett. *Breastfeeding Made Simple: Seven Natural Laws for Nursing Mothers*. Oakland: New Harbinger Publications, Inc. 2010.

Peterson, Amy, and Mindy Harmer. *Balancing Breast and Bottle: Reaching Your Breastfeeding Goals*. Hale Publishing, 2009.

Simkin, Penny. *The Birth Partner: A Complete Guide to Childbirth for Dads, Doulas, and All Other Labor Companions*. Beverly, MA: Harvard Common Press, 2007.

Wechsler-Linden, Dana. *Preemies: The Essential Guide for Parents of Premature Babies*. New York: Gallery Books, 2010.

Wiessinger, Diane. *The Womanly Art of Breastfeeding*. New York: Ballantine Books, 2010.

Zaichkin, Jeanette, ed. *Understanding the NICU: What Parents of Preemies and other Hospitalized Newborns Need to Know.* American Academy of Pediatrics, 2016.

Chapter 5: The Fourth Trimester

Johnson, Kimberly Ann. *The Fourth Trimester: A Postpartum Guide to Healing Your Body, Balancing Your Emotions, and Restoring Your Vitality.* Boulder: Shambhala Publications, 2017.

Placksin, Sally. *Mothering the New Mother.* New York: Harper Collins, 1994.

Parker, Kim. "Raising Kids and Running a Household: How Working Parents Share the Load in Close to Half of Two-Parent Families, Both Mom and Dad Work Full Time." Pew Research Center. November 4, 2015.

Vieten, Cassandra. *Mindful Motherhood: Practical Tools for Staying Sane During Pregnancy and Your Child's First Year.* Oakland: New Harbinger Publications, 2009.

Winnicott, D. W. *Babies and Their Mothers.* Cambridge: Perseus Publishing, 1987.

Wong, Kate. "Why Humans Give Birth to Helpless Babies," *Scientific American,* August 28, 2012.

Chapter 6: The First Year of Motherhood

Barha, Cindy K., and Liisa A. M. Galea. "The maternal 'baby brain' revisited," *Nature Neuroscience*, 20 (2017), 134–35.

Beebe, Beatrice. *The Mother-Infant Interaction Picture Book.* New York: W. W. Norton & Company, 2016.

Bowlby, John. *A Secure Base: Parent-Child Attachment and Healthy Human Development.* London: Routledge, 1988.

Brazelton, T. *Touchpoints: Your Child's Emotional and Behavioral Development.* Cambridge: Perseus Books, 1992.

Brody, Lauren Smith. *The Fifth Trimester: The Working Mom's Guide to Style, Sanity, and Success After Baby.* New York: Doubleday, 2017.

Chira, Susan. *A Mother's Place: Taking the Debate About Working Mothers Beyond Guilt and Blame.* New York: Harper, 1998.

Dubief, Alexis. *Precious Little Sleep: The Complete Baby Sleep Guide for Modern Parents.* Lomhara Press, 2017.

Ferber, Richard. *Solve Your Child's Sleep Problems.* New York: Touchstone, 1985.

Fernando, Nimali. *Raising a Healthy, Happy Eater: A Parent's Handbook: A*

Stage-by-Stage Guide to Setting Your Child on the Path to Adventurous Eating. The Experiment, 2015.

Hartley, Gemma. "Women Aren't Nags—We're Just Fed Up," *Harper's Bazaar*, September 27, 2017.

Karen, Robert. *Becoming Attached: First Relationships and How They Shape Our Capacity to Love.* Oxford: Oxford University Press, 1994.

Karp, Harvey. *The Happiest Baby on the Block: The New Way to Calm Crying and Help Your Newborn Baby Sleep Longer.* New York: Random House, 2002.

Le Billion, Karen. *French Kids Eat Everything.* New York: HarperCollins, 2012.

Macdonald, Cameron Lynne. *Shadow Mothers: Nannies, Au Pairs, and the Micropolitics of Mothering.* Berkeley: University of California Press, 2010.

Purvis, Karyn, David Cross, and Wendy Lyons Sunshine. *The Connected Child: Bring Hope and Healing to Your Adoptive Family.* New York: McGraw-Hill. 2007.

Rosswood, Eric. *The Ultimate Guide for Gay Dads: Everything You Need to Know About LGBTQ Parenting But Are (Mostly) Afraid to Ask.* Coral Gables, FL: Mango Publishing, 2017.

Rowell, Katja. *Helping Your Child with Extreme Picky Eating: A Step-by-Step Guide for Overcoming Selective Eating, Food Aversion, and Feeding Disorders.* New York: New Harbinger Publications, 2015.

Sacks, Alexandra. "Reframing 'Mommy Brain,'" *The New York Times*, May 11, 2018.

———. "When the Nanny Leaves," *The New York Times*, August 21, 2017.

Shortall, Jessica. *Work. Pump. Repeat.: The New Mom's Survival Guide to Breastfeeding and Going Back to Work.* New York: Abrams Books, 2015.

Appendix: Baby Blues, Postpartum Depression, and Antidepressants During Pregnancy and Breastfeeding

Abdollahi, Fatemeh, Lye Munn-Sann, Mehran Zarghami. "Perspective of Postpartum Depression Theories: A Narrative Literature Review," *North American Journal of Medical Sciences*, 8:6 (2016), 232–36.

Angelotta, and Wisner, K. L. C. "Treating Depression During Pregnancy: Are We Asking the Right Questions?," *Birth Defects Research*, 109:12 (2017), 879–87.

Bergink, V., N. Rasgon, and K. Wisner. "Postpartum Psychosis: Madness, Mania, and Melancholia in Motherhood," *American Journal of Psychiatry*, 172:12 (2016), 1179–188.

Birndorf, C., and A. Sacks. "Perinatal Mood Disorders: To Treat or Not to Treat," in Susan Dowd Stone and Alexis E. Menken, eds. *Perspectives on Perinatal Mood Disorders: A Comprehensive Treatment Guide.* New York: Springer Publishers, 2008.

Blehar, M. C., C. Spong, C. Grady, et al. "Enrolling Pregnant Women: Issues in Clinical Research." *Women's Health Issues*, 23:1 (2013), 39–45.

Cohen, L.S., L. L. Altshuler, B. L. Harlow, et al. "Relapse of Major Depression During Pregnancy in Women Who Maintain or Discontinue Anti-Depressant Treatment." *Journal of the American Medical Association*, 296:2 (2006), 170.

Fisher, S. D., K. L. Wisner, C. T. Clark, et al. "Factors Associated with Onset Timing, Symptoms and Severity of Depression Identified in the Postpartum Period." *Journal of Affective Disorders*, 203 (2016), 111–20.

Fitelson, E., S. Kim, Scott A. Baker, and K. Leight. "Treatment of Postpartum Depression: Clinical, Psychological and Pharmacological Options." *International Journal of Womens Health*, 3 (2011), 1–14.

Kleiman, Karen R. *The Postpartum Husband: Practical Solutions for Living with Postpartum Depression.* Bloomington, IN: Xlibris, 2000.

Liu, Katherine, and Natalie Mager. "Women's Involvement in Clinical Trials: Historical Perspective and Future Implications." *Pharmacy Practice.* 14:1 (2016), 708.

Miller, Laura J. *Postpartum Mood Disorders.* Washington, D.C.: American Psychiatric Publication Inc, 1999.

Miniati, M., Callari, A., Calugi, S., et al. "Interpersonal Psychotherapy for Postpartum Depression: A Systematic Review." *Archives of Women's Mental Health*, 17: 4 (2014), 257–68.

Nonacs, Ruta. *A Deeper Shade of Blue: A Woman's Guide to Recognizing and Treating Depression in Her Childbearing Years.* New York: Simon & Schuster, 2006.

Norhayati, M. N., Hazlina, N. H., Asrenee, A. R., Emilin, W. M. "Magnitude and Risk Factors for Postpartum Symptoms: A Literature Review." *Journal of Affective Disorders*, 175 (2015), 34–52.

Payne, J. L. "Psychopharmacology in Pregnancy and Breastfeeding." *Psychiatr Clinics of North America*, 40:2 (2017), 217–38.

Paulson, James F., D. Sharnail, and M. S. Bazemore. "Prenatal and Postpartum Depression in Fathers and Its Association with Maternal Depression: A Meta-analysis." *JAMA*, 303:19 (2010), 1961–69.

Puryear, Lucy J. *Understanding Your Moods When You're Expecting: Emotions, Mental Health, and Happiness—Before, During, and After Pregnancy.* New York: Houghton Mifflin, 2007.

Raskin, Valerie. *When Words Are Not Enough.* New York: Broadway Books, 1997.

Saxbe, Darby. "Postpartum Depression Can Affect Dads." *Scientific American,* August 26, 2017.

Schiller, C. E., S. Meltzer-Brody, and D. R. Rubinow. "The Role of Reproductive Hormones in Postpartum Depression." *CNS Spectrums,* 20:1 (2015), 48–59.

Sockol, L. E. "A Systematic Review of the Efficacy of Cognitive Behavioral Therapy for Treating and Preventing Perinatal Depression." *Journal of Affective Disorders,* 177 (2015), 7–21.

Stuart, S. and H. Koleva. "Psychological Treatments for Perinatal Depression." *Best Practice & Research Clinical Obstetrics & Gynaecology,* 28:1 (2014), 61–70.

Viktorin, A., S. Meltzer-Brody, R. Luja-Halkova, et al. "Heritability of Perinatal Depression and Genetic Overlap with Nonperinatal Depression." *American Journal of Psychiatry,* 173:2 (2016), 158–65.

Weissbluth, Marc. *Healthy Sleep Habits, Happy Child.* New York: Ballantine Books, 1987.

Wiegartz, Pamela. *The Pregnancy and Postpartum Anxiety Workbook.* Oakland: New Harbinger Publications, 2009.

Index

human chorionic gonadotropin (HCG), 30, 149

labor and delivery, 149–151

"nesting urge," 116

oxytocin, 31, 150, 244, 262, 292

postpartum depression and, 335

postpartum period, 149–151, 174, 175–176

progesterone, 30, 149

prolactin, 150, 262

"runner's high," 151

sexual desire and, 75

"stress hormones," 151

hospital

anxiety about baby's safety, 172–173

need for neonatal intensive care unit (NICU), 173–177

hospital tours, 131–132

human chorionic gonadotropin (HCG), 30, 149

husband/partner

"babymoon" in second trimester, 78–79

birth and, 137–143

communication skills, 211–213

depression, 338–340

dynamic with his parents, 224

infidelity, 296

as labor coach, 138–139

postpartum depression in, 338–340

in postpartum period, 208–211

reaction to pregnancy, 5–8

reconnecting with, 79

resources, 344

separation from baby, 235–236

sex during pregnancy, 75–77

sex life, 291–297

support, 338–340

supportive co-parenting, 214–216

hypervigilance, 315

idealization, 41

identity, change in pregnancy, 81–88

in-laws

advice from, 98

postpartum visits by, 221–222

presence during labor and delivery, 146

returning to work vs. stay-at-home mothering, 271–272

telling about pregnancy, 14

in vitro fertilization (IVF), 32–33

incubator, in NICU, 174

infertility. *See* fertility

insight-oriented therapy, 331

insulin, 31

Internet, as source of information, 26–27

interpersonal therapy (IPT), 83–88, 91, 93, 332

intimacy

"babymoon" in second trimester, 78

oxytocin and, 31, 292

irritability, 18–19, 31, 149, 312

isolation, following miscarriage, 23

jealousy, of older child, 238

job. *See* career/work

journaling, for stress management, 257

"kangaroo care," 174

Karp, Harvey, 253

labor and delivery, 119–179

acute stress reaction to, 161

baby sleeping in hospital nursery in first days, 171–173

birth plan, 126, 127–128, 133–137

birthing classes, 132–133

complications, 162

coping with disappointment about, 155–156

coping with traumatic delivery, 158–162

coping with upsetting feelings after, 157–158

doula, 142

emotionally processing childbirth, 154–161

emotions of, 121–123, 149–161

family and visitors, 143–148

fears about, 122–130

Acknowledgments

We are so grateful for the village that helped to birth this book. To our agents, David Kuhn and Lauren Sharp, thank you for believing in this project and finding our phenomenal editor Priscilla Painton, who, alongside Megan Hogan, brought vision, perseverance, and heart to help us shape this book so that it would help the most people. Thank you to our writing/editing assistants, Jaime Green, Ester Bloom, Sydny Miner, and Sonia Leticia Sanchez, who each brought tremendous talent, craft, and effort. And to Kimothy Joy, whose illustrations bring heart to this book and to women around the world.

To our families: Catherine wishes to thank her husband, Dan, her greatest supporter, and her daughters, Hannah and Phoebe, her greatest teachers. Alexandra wishes to thank Jeffery, Jill, Liza, Eric, and Judy. Without your love, wisdom, teaching, generosity, inspiration, and sacrifices, none of this would be possible.

To our communities that housed the production of this book in body and soul: The Motherhood Center of New York; the Columbia University Center for Psychoanalytic Training and Research; the Payne Whitney Women's Program, New York–Presbyterian/Cornell; the Columbia Women's Program at the Columbia University Medical Center; the DeWitt Wallace Institute for the History of Psychiatry, Women's Mental Health Consortium; Focus Group Women; Lady Boss Collective; Postpartum Support International; the Icahn School of Medicine at Mount Sinai Humanities and Medicine Program; TED Residency; NeuWrite; and Gimlet Media.

And finally, to the army of friends and colleagues who volunteered their time in editing, advising, researching, supporting, and sharing their stories, we feel so lucky to have you in our work and in our lives: Francesca Abbracciamento, Ruthie Ackerman, Genevieve Allen, Margaret Altemus, Cara Angelotta, Aurelie Athan, Allie Baker, Rosemary Balsam, Meg Barboza, Nathan Bashaw, Sunny Bates, Paige Bellenbaum, Wendy Belzburg, Robin Berman, Jennifer Bernstein, Carole Birndorf, Larry Birndof, Steve Birndorf, Kathryn Bleiberg, Ariane de Bonvoisin, Amber Bravo, Tracy Brenner, Mandy Brill, Louann Brizendine, Lauren Smith Brody, Marilyn Brookwood, Tony Burbank, Clare S. Burke, Christy Turlington Burns,

Bruce and Tina Buschel, Allison Carmen, Deborah Carver, Sabrina Cherry, Susan Chira, Natasha Chriss, Logan Clare, Erica Chidi Cohen, Lee Cohen, Jana Colton, Katrina Conanan, Sarah Cutler, Nicole Daily, Lucy Danziger, Seth Stephens Davidowitz, Lauren DeMille, Marissa DeVito, Heidi Dolnick, Alison Donnelly, Molly Donahue, Nehama Dresner, Lee Eisenberg, Carolyn Farnsworth, Kelly Farnsworth, Esther Fein, Kimmy Ferry, Caitlin Fiss, Elizabeth Fitelson, Sylvia Fogel, Meredith Fontecchio, Suzanne Garfinkle, Susie Gelbron, Dorian Goldman, Katja Goldman, Jennifer Goldstein, Jessica Grose, Gross Family, Jane Gross, Geoff Halber, Jennifer Halper, Ami Hamilton, Courtney Hamilton, James Hare, Cathy Harris, Amy Henderson, Alison Hermann, Margaret Howard, Tiffany Hyde, Nora Hymowitz, Lisa Inberg, Goldman-Israelow family, Mona Jain, Andrew Jenks, Kimberly Ann Johnson, Olivia Joly, Alissa Kahn, Rosy Kalfus, Harvey Karp, Justine Karp, Rebecca Kennedy, Honora Kerr, Ed Klaris, Karen Kleiman, Julie Klein, Susan Kolod, Lexie Komisar, Nathan Kravis, Jon Kurland, Roz Labow, Jackie Levin, Kate Lieb, Stacy Lindau, George Makari, Zosia Mamet, Sasha Mann, Jason Manoharan, Marcella Frydman Manoharan, Nicole Marra, Ilene Marshall, Alex Marson, Alene Mathurin, Sarah Schur McCarty, Cheryl McGibbon, Sarah McVeigh, Danielle Meister, Juliette Melton, Michelle Merrill, Catherine Monk, Rachel Moranis, Wendy N. Moyal, Kat Mustatea, Joanna Neborsky, Bruce Nichols, Morgan Nichols, Mallay Occhiogrosso, Sharone Ornstein, Lauren Osborne, Andy Parker, Lauren Pearlman, Esther Perel, Lee Perlman, Abigail Pogrebin, Robin Pogrebin, Nazanin Rafsanjani,

Acknowledgments

Christine Ragasa, Annie Rana, Erin Reade, Nicole Regent, David Remnick, Sonya Rhodes, Justin Richardson, Georgeanna Robinson, Lena Eson Roe, Alicia Rojas, Elisabeth Rosenthal, Rebekah Rosler, Gretchen Rubin, Diane H. Saran, Kate Schaffer, Laura Schiller, Brigid Schulte, Monique Scott, Selin Semaan, Karen Shike, Alexandra Snyder, Carly Snyder, Rebecca Soffer, Mariam Sologashvili, Goldman-Sonnenfeldt family, Margaret Spinelli, Shelley Stein, Seth Stephens Davidowicz, Cindi Stivers, Annie-Rose Strasser, Maya Stowe, Marianna Strongin, Devon Taylor, Cheryl Terwilliger, Tracy family, Nishi Unger, Maya Uppaluru, Susan Vaughan, Ellen Vora, Josh Weiselberg, Renee Welner, Kristen Wesley, and Roberta Zeff.

About the Authors

Alexandra Sacks, MD, is a reproductive psychiatrist affiliated with the Women's Program at the Columbia University Medical Center and a candidate at the Columbia University Psychoanalytic Center for Training and Research. A leading expert in "matrescence," she is known for popularizing the concept in her TED talk with more than one million views worldwide, and in her *New York Times* article "The Birth of a Mother," the number-one most read piece of 2017 for the "Well Family" section, where she is a regular contributor. Dr. Sacks was a scholar at the DeWitt Wallace Institute for the History of Psychiatry and serves on the American Psychoanalytic Association advisory board for media education. Her work on matrescence and "mommy brain" has been featured in *TIME* magazine, *The Washington Post*, *The Boston Globe*, and on NPR. Dr. Sacks hosts a motherhood podcast from Gimlet Media. Learn more at AlexandraSacksMD.com and @AlexandraSacksMD.

Catherine Birndorf, MD, is a reproductive psychiatrist and clinical associate professor of psychiatry at NewYork-Presbyterian/Weill Cornell Medical Center, where she founded the Payne Whitney Women's Program. She is currently the co-founder and medical director of The Motherhood Center, a treatment center in New York City for pregnant and new moms experiencing anxiety and depression. Dr. Birndorf is a board member of Postpartum Support International, a nonprofit organization for awareness, prevention, and treatment of maternal mental health worldwide. For ten years, Dr. Birndorf was a regular mental health columnist for *Self* magazine and has appeared on numerous television programs including the *TODAY* show, *Good Morning America*, *CBS Evening News*, and CNN. Her first book, *The Nine Rooms of Happiness*, co-authored with Lucy Danziger, was a *New York Times* bestseller published in 2010. Learn more at www.drcatherinebirndorf.com and www.themotherhoodcenter.com.